Physical Agents
Theory and Practice
Laboratory Manual

Second Edition

Barbara J. Behrens, PTA, MS
Coordinator, Physical Therapist Assistant Program
Mercer County Community College
Trenton, New Jersey

F. A. DAVIS COMPANY · Philadelphia

F. A. Davis Company
1915 Arch Street
Philadelphia, PA 19103

Printed in the United States of America

Last digit indicates print number: 10 9 8 7 6 5 4 3 2 1

Publisher: Margaret Biblis
Developmental Editor: Jennifer Pine
Developmental and Production Services: Molly Connors, Dovetail Content Solutions

As new scientific information becomes available through basic and clinical research, recommended treatments and drug therapies undergo changes. The author an d publisher have done everything possible to make this book accurate, up to date, and in accord with accepted standards at the time of publication. The author, editors, and publisher are not responsible for errors or omissions or for consequences from application of the book, and make no warranty, expressed or implied, in regard to the contents of the book. Any practice described in this book should be applied by the reader in accordance with professional standards of care used in regard to the unique circumstances that may apply in each situation. The reader is advised always to check product information (package inserts) for changes and new information regarding dose and contraindications before administering any drug. Caution is especially urged when using new or infrequently ordered drugs.

ISBN 13: 978-0-8036-1135-1

ISBN 10: 0-8036-1135-8

Preface

Physical agents that are used to accomplish therapeutic treatment goals are capable of causing great fear by the mere thought of their use by some clinicians. The activities in this text, as in the first edition, are designed to provide student/learners with the opportunity to experience each of the physical agents first hand, ask and answer pertinent questions regarding their application, and explore patient scenarios to help foster a greater comfort level and understanding.

Each lab activity is introduced with a purpose, objectives, and equipment needed, as well as precautions and contraindications and the rationales for each. The intent is to foster discussion and greater understanding of these important issues which are part of the decision-making process in selecting a particular physical agent to accomplish a treatment goal. Patient scenarios are included to provide opportunities for thoughtful dialogue between instructors and student/learners—for many individuals, where some of the best learning opportunities occur.

The accomplishment of therapeutic treatment goals with physical agents is an art and a science that takes time and understanding to master. These activities are intended to foster further development of the application of the science, help dispel the fears, and hopefully lead to a greater appreciation of what potentially can be accomplished with a sound physiological rationale.

Barbara J. Behrens, PTA, MS

Acknowledgments

Being involved in publishing is somewhat of a thankless task for those who are involved in the production side of putting together the work that the author has written, except when someone reads the acknowledgements in a book.

Along the way, there have been many hands and minds involved in putting this project together whom I would like to thank, including Jean-François Villain, Margaret Biblis, and Jennifer Pine of F. A. Davis Company and Molly Connors of Dovetail Content Solutions. Each of these individuals has had to put up with deadlines, revisions, and periodic "meetings of the minds" to help bring this book together. Thank you.

Thank you to the reviewers who lent their time and expertise to help me put together a more cohesive version of what I had envisioned.

Thank you to my parents who have continued to encourage my seemingly endless desire to "do more" and who have understood when I have been swamped because of it.

Thanks to the student/learners in the PTA program at MCCC who have patiently worked through the revision process and tolerated it well.

Thanks to Mel for always being by my side, even when I fall asleep while working late on projects like this one.

Reviewers

Susan Callanan, DPT
Assistant Instructor
Physical Therapy Department
North Iowa Area Community College
Mason City, Iowa

Elizabeth A. Chape, PT, MS
Program Coordinator
Physical Therapy Assistant Program
Science and Allied Health Department
Sacramento City College
Sacramento, California

Martha R. Hinman, PT, EdD
Professor
Physical Therapy Department
Hardin-Simmons University
Abilene, Texas

Marlene Medin, PT, MEd
Program Director
Physical Therapy Assistant Program
Linn State Technical College
Linn, Missouri

Therese Millis, PT
Professor
Physical Therapy Department
San Juan College
Farmington, New Mexico

Sidney Morgan
Physical Therapist Assistant
Allied Health and Physical Therapy Assistant Department
Northeastern Oklahoma A&M College
Miami, Oklahoma

Maria M. Pappas, PT
Associate Professor
Physical Therapy Assistant Department
MassBay Community College
Framingham, Massachusetts

James K. Tenpenny, AAS
Associate Professor
Physical Therapy Assistant Program
Kaskaskia College
Centralia, Illinois

Frank B. Underwood, PT, PhD, ECS
Professor
Physical Therapy Department
University of Evansville
Evansville, Indiana

Peter Zawicki, PT, MS
Program Chair
Physical Therapy Assistant Program
Department of Health Sciences
Gateway Community College
Phoenix, Arizona

Contents

Tissue Response to Injury

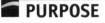

1

PURPOSE

These lab activities provide student/learners with the opportunity to review tissue response concepts that may have been presented previously in other courses.

OBJECTIVES

Following the completion of this lab activity, the student/learner will be able to:

- Define the following terms that are commonly used in the clinical setting to describe symptoms related to tissue responses
  - pain
  - altered sensation
  - edema (swelling)
  - loss of function
- Describe the common concepts for the theory of pain transmission and perception and explain it in terms that a patient would understand
- Describe the similarities and differences between the endogenous opiates in terms that a patient would understand
- Discuss the impact of the psychological component on pain perception by comparing his or her findings and experiences with those of classmates in a guided class discussion
- Discuss a classic theory of pain transmission and how it can be applied to pain-relieving techniques
- Differentiate between the key events in the three stages of wound healing by describing each of those key events and what triggers them
- Describe the necessary precautions in handling wounds during each of the stages of healing

LAB ACTIVITIES

Pain

1. Look up the definition of pain in three dictionaries and develop a composite definition that encompasses all of them.

   Source/Definition: _____

   _____

   Source/Definition: _____

   _____

   Source/Definition: _____

   _____

Composite Definition: _____

_____

_____

2. How much of the definition was based on psychological factors and how much on physical factors?

Psychological Factors: _____

Physical Factors: _____

3. How could this potentially be useful information for you as a clinician?

_____

_____

_____

_____

4. Look up and write down the definitions of analgesia, anesthesia, and paresthesia.

Analgesia: _____

Anesthesia: _____

Paresthesia: _____

5. What is the difference between the three?

_____

_____

• Which would be a symptom of more concern?

_____

_____

• Why?

_____

_____

Edema

1. Review your definitions for edema or look it up again and write it below.

_____

_____

_____

_____

2. Based on the definition that you have written, how would edema potentially limit function?

_____

_____

_____

_____

3. What would you consider to be a reliable indicator of the amount of edema present? Why?

_____

_____

_____

_____

Pain Transmission

1. Review your text and describe why sensory input to an intact peripheral nerve is capable of providing pain relief in the same location on the opposite side of the body.

_____

_____

_____

_____

Endogenous Opiates

1. What are the differences between enkephalin and beta-endorphin?

_____

_____

_____

_____

2. If it is possible to stimulate the liberation of one or both of the listed endogenous opiates, which would be more difficult to stimulate?

_____

_____

_____

_____

3. What pharmacologic agents potentially inhibit the liberation of the longer-lasting endogenous opiates?

_____

_____

_____

_____

Psychology and Pain

1. Interview three people of different ethnic groups and generations to find out how they would describe the pain associated with each of the following stimuli:

	First Individual	Second Individual	Third Individual
A severe sunburn			
Overexposure to sub-freezing temperatures			
Hitting a thumb with a hammer			
An extremity that "falls asleep"			

2. Compare the sensation descriptions that you have solicited. Are there any differences in reported responses that surprised you? Why or why not?

_____

_____

_____

_____

3. What practical knowledge could you gain from this activity?

_____

_____

_____

_____

4. Providing sensory stimulation to an area will decrease the perception of painful stimuli in that area.

- What response from your interviewees supports this theory?

  _____

  _____

  _____

- What is the name of this theory, first described in 1965 by Melzack and Wall?

  _____

  _____

  _____

- How can this information be applied practically today?

  _____

  _____

  _____

Stages of Wound Healing

1. What are the three stages of wound/tissue healing, and approximately how long does each stage last?

First: _____

_____

Second: _____

_____

Third: _____

_____

2. What is the primary purpose for each of the stages, and what is the indicator for whether or not that stage of healing is occurring?

Stage	Purpose	Indicator
First		
Second		
Third		

Precautions in Handling Wounds in Each Stage

1. Each of the stages of wound/tissue healing involves a significant number of activities. Wound/tissue healing is vulnerable to potential "setbacks" that could delay the healing process. Review your texts for examples of precautions that may adversely affect this process.

First: _____

_____

Second: _____

_____

Third: _____

_____

◼ LAB QUESTIONS

1. What have you learned from the activities in this lab exercise about tissue responses to injury?
2. Do all patients respond the same way to the same types of stimuli? Why or why not?
3. What types of factors tend to influence the way that a patient responds to "painful stimuli?"
4. How will the responses that you noted from your classmates influence your expectations for patient responses in the future?

Patient Responses to Therapeutic Interventions

2

PURPOSE

These lab activities are designed to emphasize the importance of observational skills for patient responses to therapeutic interventions and to lay the foundation for problem solving. Throughout these lab activities, student/learners will be instructed to apply several different forms of thermal agents that are commonly used in the clinic and note each patient's responses. In performing these, student/learners will discover that there are a variety of responses and application techniques. In the course of these activities, student/learners are expected to position and drape their patients appropriately, practice principles of safe body mechanics, observe patient responses, and share the responsibility of being both the clinician and the patient.

OBJECTIVES

Following the completion of this lab activity, the student/learner will be able to:

- Describe and identify expected responses to the application of superficial heat and cold
- Provide the rationale for skin assessment before and after the application of physical agents to the skin by demonstrating the techniques on a classmate
- Differentiate between normal and abnormal responses to heat and cold as observed in a controlled activity with classmates
- Document observations of skin appearance of a classmate in terms that would be appropriate for a patient record
- Note the similarities and differences in normal responses to heat and cold by applying both to classmates and noting their individual responses
- Integrate the problem-solving process for determining techniques for applying cold by comparing several application techniques and discussing the outcomes
- Describe the sequence of sensations associated with the application of heat and cold through personal experience with a variety of examples of heat and cold as applied by a classmate

EQUIPMENT THAT YOU WILL NEED

towels	minute timer	ice cubes
hot packs	water basin	thermometer (high and low temps)
ice packs	pillow cases	

◼ PRECAUTIONS AND WHY

Precaution	Why?
Past experience with the agent	It is always helpful to solicit this information from a patient. It will guide you in determining whether a previous attempt with this intervention was successful or not and whether any adverse responses were experienced. It will also help to establish a rapport with the patient with regard to their expectations for an intervention.
Open wounds	Fresh granulated tissue is too fragile for the application of many physical agents; however, proximal application techniques may enhance circulation to healing areas.
Peripheral vascular disease	If there is a diagnosed difficulty with circulation to the lower extremity, a proximal application technique of a thermal agent may exacerbate lower extremity discomfort.
Advanced age	Older patients may have less adipose or connective tissue to insulate them against extremes of heat or cold. This may make them more susceptible to burns. In addition, their superficial layer of skin is often thinner and more fragile.
Pregnancy	Application of heat or cold directly over a pregnant uterus is contraindicated; however, application to other areas of the body is not.
Impaired cognitive ability	If a patient is unable to communicate discomfort, application of heat or cold would be contraindicated; however, if they have cognitive limitations but are able to provide this information and their skin blanches appropriately, the intervention may be undertaken with precaution.
Metastases	Application of heat or cold directly over a metastasis is contraindicated, because it could potentially increase circulation to the area. However, if the malignancy is terminal and the patient has found heat or cold to be beneficial as a palliative treatment, it may be applied with caution. Special care should be taken to ensure that nerve roots to distally related areas are NOT treated with heat, because they may increase circulation to the metastasized area.

◼ CONTRAINDICATIONS AND WHY

Contraindication	Heat	Cold	Why?
Unreliable patient responses	X	X	The patient may burn or develop frostbite without warning.
Anti-coagulant medications	X		The patient may experience hyperemia easily and be unable to regulate their temperature.

Contraindication	Heat	Cold	Why?
Metastasis in the treatment area	X	X	An increase in circulation may enhance the spread of the malignancy.
Absence of sensation in the treatment area	X	X	The patient may burn or develop frostbite without warning.
Frostbite in the treatment area	X	X	The patient may have an inability to adapt to sudden temperature changes, and application of heat or cold may be extremely painful.
Peripheral vascular disease distal to the treatment area	X		Heat may produce a local increase in circulation which would exacerbate patient discomfort rather than relieve it.
Acute inflammation	X		Heat could exacerbate the inflammatory response, causing further bleeding and potentially inducing shock.
Deep vein thrombosis	X		Heat would exacerbate the inflammatory response in an area that cannot accommodate circulatory changes. A clot could potentially dislodge and travel to the heart, lungs, or brain.
Acute hemorrhage	X		Heat would exacerbate the inflammatory response and increase discomfort.
Fever	X		Heat would exacerbate the inflammatory response and increase discomfort.
Over a pregnant uterus during the first trimester	X	X	There is no indication for this application. Studies have not been performed to show the effects on the fetus to determine whether or not it would be detrimental.

LAB ACTIVITIES

ASSESSMENT TECHNIQUES

- **Observation of Skin Types and Responses**

1. Select two classmates/patients who have different skin types and list them below. Record your observations of their knees in terms of skin type, location of any visible scars (noting the age and condition of each), and ability to differentiate among heat, cold, light touch, dull touch, sharp touch, and pain.

Name (Classmate/Patient)	Scars	Sensation

- **Observation of Joint Range of Motion in Response to Heat**

- **Observation of Scar Tissue in Response to Superficial Heat Application**

Application of Superficial Heat

1. Position both patients so that each is supine with his or her knees supported in about 10 to 20 degrees of flexion by placing a towel roll, pillow, or bolster underneath his or her knees (Fig. 2-1).

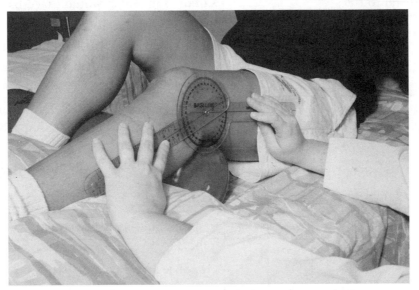

Figure 2-1 Patient is positioned so that the knee is in approximately 20 degrees of flexion, after the skin has been inspected for scars and sensation.

2. Remove two standard size hot packs from the hydrocollator unit. Wrap one hot pack in toweling so that there will be 4 layers of towel between the hot pack and the patient (Fig. 2-2). Wrap the second hot pack in toweling so that there will be 6 layers between the patient and the hot pack. *(Use only towels, not commercial covers, for this exercise.)*

3. Record the following information while the hot packs are on the patients' knees.

Patient 1 (4 Layers)	At 3 Minutes	At 6 Minutes	At 9 Minutes	At 12 Minutes
Appearance under the pack				
Patient report of "how it feels"				

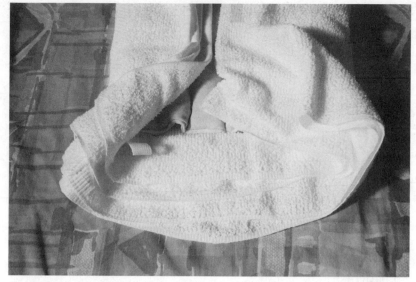

Figure 2-2 Standard size hot pack has been removed from the Hydrocollator unit and placed on 2 towels that have been folded in half, providing 4 layers of towel between the patient and the pack.

Patient 2 (6 Layers)	At 3 Minutes	At 6 Minutes	At 9 Minutes	At 12 Minutes
Appearance under the pack				
Patient report of "how it feels"				

4. Remove the hot packs from the patients and observe the knees again, recording any differences in appearance and sensation from that which you observed before the hot pack application. Place the hot packs in the hydrocollator unit for reuse.

	Change in Appearance	Change in Sensation
Patient 1 (4 layers)		
Patient 2 (6 layers)		

Patient's Observations Regarding His or Her "Heated Knee"

1. Ask the patients to get up and walk around. Observe their gaits, and ask each to describe how the treated knee feels as he or she walks on it.

	Patient 1 (4 Layers)	Patient 2 (6 Layers)
How does the "heated knee" feel? (tight, loose, etc.)		
Is there symmetry in the gait?		
Were there any differences between the perceptions of the two patients?		

2. How would you describe what you observed when you looked at the patient's knee after the hot pack had been applied for 6 minutes?

   • Was there any uniformity to what you observed?
   • Why or why not?

   Patient 1 (4 Layers): _____

   _____

   Patient 2 (6 Layers): _____

   _____

3. If the patient had any scars, did the scar tissue respond the same way as the non-scarred or uninvolved tissue?

   Patient 1 (4 Layers): _____

   _____

   Patient 2 (6 Layers): _____

   _____

4. How would the presence of a scar in the treatment area potentially affect your treatment?

   _____

   _____

   _____

   _____

5. Why is the age of the scar significant?

_____

_____

_____

_____

6. What would you expect to see if the patient had a recent (4 weeks post-op) meniscectomy scar on the medial aspect of the knee?

Patient 1 (4 Layers): _____

_____

Patient 2 (6 Layers): _____

_____

7. What would you expect to see if the patient had a knee replacement 2 years ago?

Patient 1 (4 Layers): _____

_____

Patient 2 (6 Layers): _____

_____

8. Which patient did you expect to potentially feel the heat sooner?

_____

_____

9. How long after you had applied the hot packs did the patients report that the level of heat had plateaued?

_____ 3 minutes   _____ 9 minutes

_____ 6 minutes   _____ 12 minutes

10. In the future, how would you decide whether or not a patient should have 4 or 6 layers of towels?

_____

_____

_____

_____

11. How long would you expect the effects from the hot pack to last? (How long did it take before the patients' knees returned to their pretreatment appearance?)

Patient 1 (4 Layers): _____

_____

Patient 2 (6 Layers): _____

_____

12. Based on the patients' responses to how their knees felt when walking after the hot pack application, how, if at all, would this impact your instructions to future patients?

_____

_____

_____

_____

ASSESSMENT TECHNIQUES

- ### Observation of Range of Motion in Response to Cold

1. Select three classmates/patients to receive ice packs on their cervical spine and cervical musculature. They should be patients who have demonstrable tightness in their upper trapezius muscles, preferably with palpable nodules in the musculature.

2. Observe their available range of motion (ROM) and record your findings in the table below.

3. Palpate any nodules and ask the patient to rate their discomfort on a scale of 1 to 10, where 1 is minimal discomfort and 10 is maximal discomfort. Record your findings in the table below.

4. Stretch the upper trapezius bilaterally and note the patient response to the stretch and ease of movement during the stretch. Record your findings in the table on the next page.

	Patient 1	Patient 2	Patient 3
Cervical ROM			
Any palpable nodules?			

	Patient 1	Patient 2	Patient 3
Response to stretch			
Pain rating with stretch or pressure (1–10 scale)			

5. Position the patients so that they are supported, the cervical spine is neutral, and the postural muscles are at rest (Fig. 2-3).

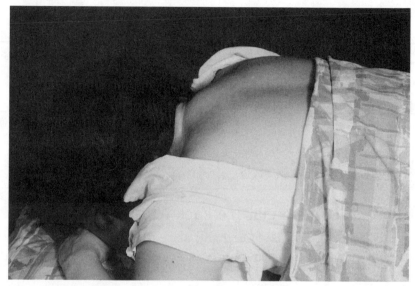

Figure 2-3 Patient positioning and draping prior to receiving commercial cold pack application to the upper trapezius. Patient is positioned to place the postural muscles at rest.

Application of a Commercial Ice Pack Directly on the Skin

1. Remove a cold pack from the freezer and place it directly on the upper trapezius, which you observed to be tight and painful for the patient.

2. Cover the area with a towel and drape the patient.

3. Observe the patient and record your observations at the intervals provided in the table below.

Patient 1 (Ice Pack Directly on Skin)	At 3 Minutes	At 6 Minutes	At 9 Minutes	At 12 Minutes
Patient response				
Skin appearance				

Patient 1 (Ice Pack Directly on Skin)	At 3 Minutes	At 6 Minutes	At 9 Minutes	At 12 Minutes
Reassessment				
Cervical ROM				
Any palpable nodules?				
Response to stretch				
Pain rating with stretch or pressure (1–10 scale)				

Application of a Commercial Ice Pack Within a Pillow Case

1. Remove a cold pack from the freezer and place it in a pillow case. Apply the covered ice pack to the upper trapezius that you observed to be tight and painful for the patient.

2. Cover the area with a towel and drape the patient.

3. Observe the patient and record your observations at the intervals provided in the table below.

Patient 2 (Ice Pack in Pillow Case)	At 3 Minutes	At 6 s Minutes	At 9 Minutes	At 12 Minutes
Patient response				
Skin appearance				
Reassessment				

Patient 2 (Ice Pack in Pillow Case)	At 3 Minutes	At 6 Minutes	At 9 Minutes	At 12 Minutes
Cervical ROM				
Any palpable nodules?				
Response to stretch				
Pain rating with stretch or pressure (1–10 scale)				

Application of a Commercial Ice Pack Within a Damp Pillow Case

1. Remove a cold pack from the freezer and place it in a dampened pillow case. Apply the covered damp pack to the upper trapezius that you observed to be tight and painful for the patient.

2. Cover the area with a towel and drape the patient.

3. Observe the patient and record your observations at the intervals provided in the table below.

Patient 3 (Ice Pack in Dampened Pillow Case)	At 3 Minutes	At 6 Minutes	At 9 Minutes	At 12 Minutes
Patient response				
Skin appearance				
Reassessment				
Cervical ROM				

Patient 3 (Ice Pack in Dampened Pillow Case)	At 3 Minutes	At 6 Minutes	At 9 Minutes	At 12 Minutes
Any palpable nodules?				
Response to stretch				
Pain rating with stretch or pressure (1–10 scale)				

LAB QUESTIONS

1. You have worked with several classmate/patients during the lab activity and applied either heat or cold to the indicated areas. What, if any, were the common visual observations that you made of the areas before and after the application of a thermal agent?
2. What preapplication observations proved to be the most important for you in determining whether to select more layers between the thermal agent and the patient? Why?
3. Based on your experiences and observations and those of your classmates, of what potential significance is the presence of a visible scar in the treatment area to receive a thermal agent?
4. If the patient was incapable of accurately reporting sensation in the proposed treatment area, how might this affect your decision-making process for this patient?
5. During the application of the thermal agents, did you find that the patient ever neglected to tell you that the sensation was too strong, resulting in an adverse response? If yes, what would you do in the future to prevent this from occurring?

Therapeutic Heat and Cold

3

PURPOSE

These lab activities involve application techniques for several therapeutic heating agents including: hydrocollator (hot) packs, paraffin, Fluidotherapy™, shortwave diathermy, and cryotherapy. Student/learners are expected to both receive and administer treatments to their classmates, recording observations from both perspectives as indicated.

The exercises are intended to allow student/learners to compare different application techniques, determine alternative treatment set-ups, learn to describe and document the sensations of different forms of therapeutic heat and cold, and begin to familiarize themselves with the similarities and differences among the thermal agents.

OBJECTIVES

Following the completion of this lab activity, the student/learner will be able to:

- Describe the normal sensations perceived in response to the application of a variety of thermal agents through having the agents applied to them by a classmate and recording the sensations. The thermal agents for this exercise include:
    - hydrocollator packs
    - paraffin
    - Fluidotherapy™
    - shortwave diathermy
    - cryotherapy
- Identify practical application techniques and challenges for thermal agents by participating in problem-solving activities in guided lab activities using physical agents.
- Integrate the problem-solving process into the application of therapeutic heat for a patient by practicing the techniques with a classmate, discussing outcomes and soliciting feedback.
- Integrate the problem-solving process into the application of therapeutic cold for a patient by practicing the techniques with a classmate, discussing outcomes and soliciting feedback.

EQUIPMENT THAT YOU WILL NEED

towels	gowns	pillows and cases
plastic bags	minute timer	hydrocollator packs (various sizes)
Fluidotherapy™	paraffin unit	shortwave diathermy
thermometer	ice cubes	ice bath
basin	ice packs	

PRECAUTIONS AND WHY

Precaution	Why?
Open wounds	New granulation tissue is sensitive to heat, cold, and pressure and may not be able to withstand heat or cold application. However, heat may enhance circulation to the area once the wound is closed. Skin sensation must be intact to administer heat or cold.
Pregnancy	Heat may be beneficial; however, it should not be applied over a pregnant uterus as it may increase the circulation to the fetus, and the effects of this have not been studied.
Advanced age	If the patient has intact sensation and is reliable, then the application of heat or cold may be indicated. However, if the patient has fragile skin that does not blanche under pressure, they may not be able to adapt to the increased temperature from application of heat.
Menses	Heat applied to the lower back or over the pelvis of a female during menses may increase menstrual flow. If she is prepared for this, then the application might be indicated depending on the signs and symptoms of the physical therapy diagnosis.
Impaired cognitive ability	If a patient is able to communicate sensations of heat, cold, and pain in some meaningful way, then they may have applied. However, these patients should be monitored closely.
Previous experience with the physical agent	If a patient has had a poor response to the application of a thermal agent in the past, they may be less receptive to trying it again. However, it is important that the clinician educate the patient and explain the potential benefits of any modality before it is applied.

CONTRAINDICATIONS AND WHY

Contra-indications	Hydrocollator Packs, Paraffin, Fluidotherapy™	Diathermy
Pregnancy (first trimester)	Heat should not be applied directly over a pregnant uterus as it may increase the circulation to the fetus and this has not been studied for safety in humans.	In addition to concerns with application of heat, the effects of electromagnetic fields on the fetus have not been studied for safety in humans.
Undressed or infected wounds	The infection must be cultured and treated first. The wound must be covered to prevent cross-contamination.	The infection must be cultured and treated first. The wound must be covered to prevent cross-contamination.

Contra-indications	Hydrocollator Packs, Paraffin, Fluidotherapy™	Diathermy
Pacemaker	If the pacemaker is a demand pacemaker, then only precautions are necessary. Application of heat in patients with non–demand-type pacemakers may cause undue stress on the cardiac musculature.	In addition to concerns with application of heat, electromagnetic energy may leak and effect the operation of the pacemaker which could be harmful to the patient.
Metastasis	Heat applied directly over or proximal to a metastasis will increase circulation to the area and may enhance the disease progression.	Heat applied directly over or proximal to a metastasis will increase circulation to to the area and may enhance the disease progression.
Fever	Heat applied to an area actively involved in the inflammatory process will result in an increase in the circulation to that area and potentially increase edema.	Heat applied to an area actively involved in the inflammatory process will result in an increase in the circulation to that area and potentially increase edema.
Acute inflammation	Heat applied to an area actively involved in the inflammatory process will result in an increase in the circulation to that area and potentially increase edema.	Heat applied to an area actively involved in the inflammatory process will result in an increase in the circulation to that area and potentially increase edema.
Acute hemorrhage	Heat applied to an area actively involved in the inflammatory process will result in an increase in the circulation to that area and potentially increase bleeding.	Heat applied to an area actively involved in the inflammatory process will result in an increase in the circulation to that area and potentially increase bleeding.
Peripheral vascular disease	Heat applied to an area with compromised ability to maintain homeostasis may result in increased pain perception and other complications.	Heat applied to an area with compromised ability to maintain homeostasis may result in increased pain perception and other complications.
Lack of sensation	The safety of heat application relies on the ability of the patient to report changes in sensation to prevent a burn.	The safety of heat application relies on the ability of the patient to report changes in sensation to prevent a burn.

Contra-indications	Hydrocollator Packs, Paraffin, Fluidotherapy™	Diathermy
Presence of metal implants or jewelry	None	The metal may significantly increase in temperature and cause a burn.
Operation of a mechanical traction unit	None	Unless the diathermy unit is shielded, the electro-magnetic energy from the diathermy may change the settings on the traction unit. Distance from the unit should be 10 feet.

◤ LAB ACTIVITIES

Hydrocollator Packs (Hot Packs)

APPLICATION TECHNIQUES

1. Select three classmates/patients who will have hot packs applied to their lower backs. You will position each of them differently to compare the conduction of thermal energy from the hot pack to each of the patients. As with all treatments, inspect the area and note the presence of scars, edema, muscle guarding, or impairment in sensation. Remember, scars may not conduct heat as uniformly as unscarred areas.

Prone

1. Position patient 1 prone with a pillow underneath his or her abdomen and ankles to reduce lordosis and permit treatment in a neutral spine position (Fig. 3-1).

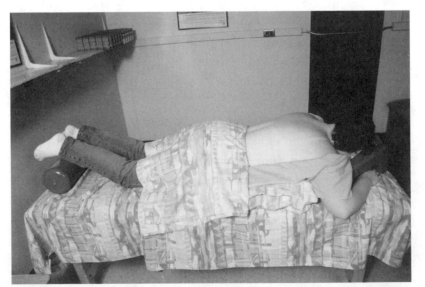

Figure 3-1 Patient positioning for application of lumbar hot pack. The sheet is draping the lumbar area in preparation for the application of heat.

2. Remove a standard size hot pack and place it in a commercial cover. Place a folded towel over the treatment area, and place the hot pack on top of the folded towel. Drape the patient.

3. Ask the patient to describe what he or she feels on the back at the intervals noted and record the descriptions in the table below.

Initially	After 5 Minutes	After 8 Minutes	After 10 Minutes

4. Did the patient ever report that the hot pack was getting too warm? If yes, after how long, and what did you do?

_____

_____

_____

_____

Supine

1. Position patient 2 so that he or she is supine, with a pillow underneath the head and knees for support. Clothing should be removed in the treatment area so that it will not be in the way of the hot pack.

2. Remove a standard size hot pack and place it in a commercial cover. Place a folded towel on top of the cover and ask the patient to lift up so that you can place the hot pack underneath him or her.

3. Ask the patient to describe what he or she feels on the back at the intervals noted and record the descriptions in the table below.

Initially	After 5 Minutes	After 8 Minutes	After 10 Minutes

4. Did the patient ever report that the hot pack was getting too warm? If yes, after how long, and what did you do?

_____

_____

_____

_____

NOTE: The supine position is NOT recommended for clinical use because it causes compression of the body weight against the hot pack. This impedes blood flow, which counteracts the desired effects of the hot pack. This also increases the skin's susceptibility to a burn.

Side Lying

1. Position patient 3 so that he or she is side lying. You will have to determine what you need to do to ensure that the hot pack is in good contact with the lumbar spine. It is important that the patient is well supported in a neutral position and is comfortable. (A wall or strap may work well.)

2. Describe the position that you decided on and indicate the rationale for your choice.

   _____

   _____

   _____

   _____

3. Remove a standard size hot pack and place it in a commercial cover. Place a folded towel over the treatment area, and place the hot pack on the folded towel. Secure the hot pack in place.

4. Ask the patient to describe what he or she feels on the back at the intervals noted and record the descriptions in the table below.

Initially	After 5 Minutes	After 8 Minutes	After 10 Minutes

5. Did the patient ever report that the hot pack was getting too warm? If yes, after how long, and what did you do?

   _____

   _____

   _____

   _____

Hydrocollator Application Questions

1. Remove the hot packs from the patients after 15 minutes, and reassess the treatment area. Leave a layer of toweling on the treatment area while you return the hot pack to the hydrocollator unit. (This will keep some of the heat and moisture from evaporating from the patient's skin.)

2. Record your observations of the patients in the table below.

	Prone	Supine	Side Lying
Subjectively, which patient initially felt the most comfortable?			
Were all 3 patients still comfortable after 10 minutes? If no, who was not, and what is your explanation for this?			
How long did it take for the heat from the hot pack to plateau for each of the patients?			
Which position was the easiest for you to add towel layers if you needed to?			
Which patient had the greatest amount of erythema after hot pack removal? Why?			
Which patient had the least amount of erythema after hot pack removal? Why?			
When would each of the positions that you tried be indicated?			
How long after hot pack removal did it take for the appearance of the treated area to return to its pretreatment appearance?			

3. What temperature was the hydrocollator unit kept at?

_____

4. Was the water level in the hydrocollator unit sufficient to cover the hot packs completely? What difference, if any, would the water level make?

_____

_____

5. There are a variety of sizes and shapes of hot packs to allow for better contouring and therefore conduction of the thermal energy of the hot pack. Try them and see what size or shape works best in the following areas of the body, and describe your patient positioning techniques in the table below.

	Hot Pack Shape/Size	Positioning
Shoulder		
Hip		
Knee		
Cervical spine		

Paraffin

APPLICATION TECHNIQUES

1. Select two classmates/patients who will each have paraffin applied to one of their hands using different methods. Inspect and wash the hands, recording any observations you make. Remember that scars or areas of decreased sensation require caution owing to the lack of uniform patient response to sensation in that area. Paraffin can be applied using several different methods. For this exercise, you will compare the dip method to the continuous immersion method.

2. What is the temperature of the paraffin unit that you will be using?

_____

3. What is the optimal treatment temperature?

_____

4. Why can patients tolerate such a high temperature without getting burned?

_____

_____

Dip Method

1. Ask the patient to dip his or her hand and wrist into the paraffin unit, remove it, and let the paraffin harden (Fig. 3-2). Then instruct them to re-dip to achieve 8 to 10 layers of paraffin (Fig. 3-3).

2. Wrap the dipped hand in plastic wrap (Figs. 3-4 and 3-5) and then in a towel (Figs. 3-6 through 3-8).

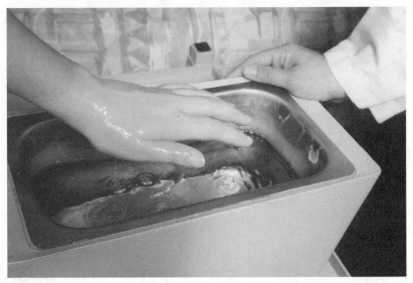

Figure 3-2 Dip method of paraffin application. After the first dip, the patient lets the wax harden before re-immersing for subsequent dips.

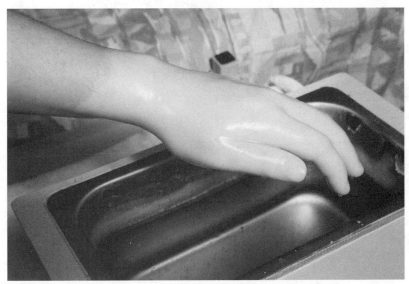

Figure 3-3 Dip method of paraffin application. The left distal upper extremity after several dips.

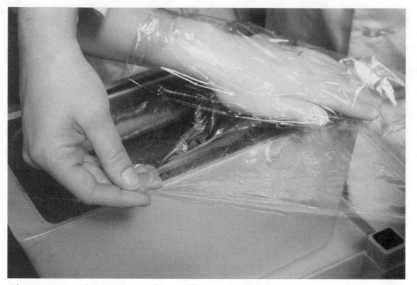

Figure 3-4 Dip method of paraffin application. Plastic wrap is wrapped around the paraffin-dipped hand.

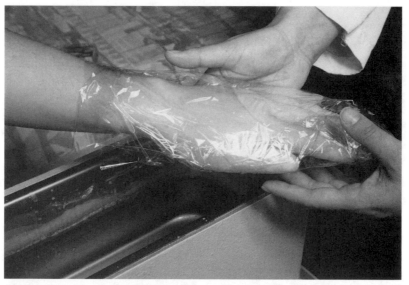

Figure 3-5 Dip method of paraffin application. Plastic wrap is secured around the paraffin-dipped hand.

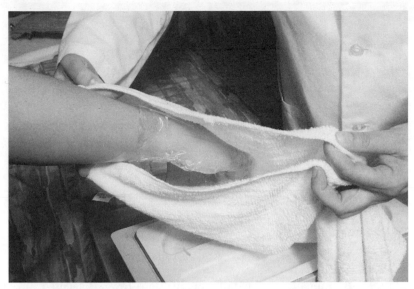

Figure 3-6 Dip method of paraffin application. Plastic-wrapped hand is inserted into a folded towel.

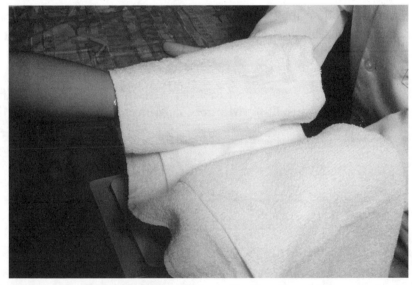

Figure 3-7 Dip method of paraffin application. Towel is wrapped around the paraffin-dipped hand.

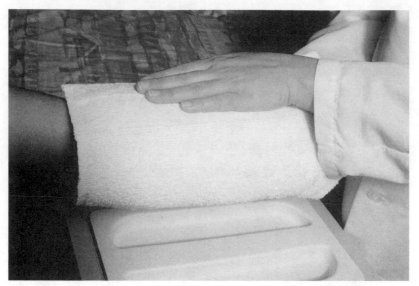

Figure 3-8 Dip method of paraffin application. Towel is secured around the paraffin-dipped hand.

3. Position the patient for a 15-minute treatment time, making sure that the dipped hand is supported and elevated above the heart.

4. Ask the patient to describe how the paraffin feels during treatment and after removal at the intervals noted and record the descriptions and your observations in the table below.

	Initially	After 3 Minutes	After 6 Minutes	After 9 Minutes	After 12 Minutes
Ask the patient to describe how the paraffin feels.					
Ask the patient to describe how his or her hand feels after the paraffin is removed.					
Reassess the patient and document your observations.					

5. The paraffin that you remove may either be manipulated in the patient's hand until it cools or removed entirely. The hand is then reassessed. Some facilities require that the paraffin be disposed of after use. Other facilities may allow return of the paraffin to the bath for re-melting.

Continuous Immersion Method

1. Ask the patient to immerse his or her hand and wrist into the paraffin unit, remove it, and let the paraffin harden. Then ask him or her to re-immerse the hand and wrist into the unit and leave it in the unit. He or she should be careful to not move their fingers or break the "glove" of paraffin that was initially formed.

2. Position the patient so that he or she will be comfortable and supported during the 15-minute immersion treatment.

3. Ask the patient to describe how the paraffin feels during treatment and after removal at the intervals noted and record the descriptions and your observations in the table below.

	Initially	After 3 Minutes	After 6 Minutes	After 9 Minutes	After 12 Minutes
Ask the patient to describe how the paraffin feels.					
Ask the patient to describe how his or her hand feels after the paraffin is removed.					
Which technique was "tolerated better" by the patient and why?					
Was the patient able to withstand the full treatment time in the paraffin unit?					
Which patients may not be able to withstand the entire treatment time? Why?					
Reassess the patient and document your observations.					

Paraffin Application Questions

1. Describe the appearance of each of the treated hands after removal from the paraffin. Is there a difference? Why or why wouldn't you expect to see one?

_____

_____

_____

_____

2. What types of patient diagnoses would potentially be better suited for each of the techniques and why?

   Dip Method: _____

   _____

   Immersion Method: _____

   _____

3. What would you do if, before immersing the patient's hand into the paraffin unit, you noted that the temperature was 140°F?

_____

_____

_____

_____

Fluidotherapy™

APPLICATION TECHNIQUES

1. Select two classmates/patients, each of whom will be immersing one of their hands into a Fluidotherapy™ unit. Inspect and wash the hands, recording any additional observations that you make. You will compare two different treatment techniques: one that is used to help promote the healing of uninfected wounds, and one that is used to provide heat and desensitization to the immersed body part.

2. What is the temperature of the Fluidotherapy™ unit?

_____

3. What is the optimal treatment temperature?

_____

4. What could you do to insure that the unit is the right temperature when you need it?

_____

_____

_____

_____

Bagged or Gloved Technique (Nonspecific Debridement of a Wound)

1. After washing and drying the patient's hand, secure it in either a plastic bag or glove so that it is airtight. Tape the bag or glove so that the edges are covered with tape that adheres to the skin. It may be necessary to use 2 plastic bags if they are thin.

2. Place the bagged hand into the media in the unit and secure the sleeve around the forearm.

3. Position the patient so that he or she will be supported and comfortable for the 10- to 12-minute treatment time.

4. Turn the unit on without any turbulence or agitation. Gradually adjust the turbulence so that it is comfortable for the patient.

5. Ask the patient to describe how his or her hand feels during treatment at the intervals noted and record the descriptions and your observations in the table below.

	Initially	After 3 Minutes	After 6 Minutes	After 9 Minutes	After 12 Minutes
Ask the patient to describe how his or her hand feels.					
Does it feel dry or damp? Does that sensation change? If yes, when?					

	Initially	After 3 Minutes	After 6 Minutes	After 9 Minutes	After 12 Minutes
Does he or she report any desire to move in the media? Can he or she?					
Reassess the patient and document your observations.					

6. Adjust the agitation in the unit so that it is different than it was during the treatment time. Ask the patient to move his or her hand again. How has this changed his or her ability to move?

_____

_____

_____

_____

7. Turn off the unit and slowly remove the patient's hand from the unit. Carefully brush the media back into the unit and secure the sleeve.

8. What is the temperature of the unit after the treatment time?

_____

Unbagged Technique (Most Commonly Applied Technique)

1. After washing and drying the hand that will be immersed in the Fluidotherapy™ unit, instruct the patient to reach into the media. Secure the sleeve of the unit so that NO media will escape during the treatment time.

2. Position the patient so that he or she will be supported and comfortable for the 12-minute treatment time.

3. Turn the unit on without any turbulence or agitation. Gradually adjust the turbulence so that it is comfortable for the patient. (Some patients prefer more agitation than others.)

4. Ask the patient to describe how his or her hand feels during treatment at the intervals noted and record the descriptions and your observations in the table below.

	Initially	After 3 Minutes	After 6 Minutes	After 9 Minutes	After 12 Minutes
Ask the patient to describe how his or her hand feels.					
Does it feel dry or damp? Does that sensation change? If yes, when?					
Does he or she report any desire to move in the media? Can he or she?					
Reassess the patient and document your observations.					

5. Adjust the agitation in the unit so that it is different than it was during the treatment time. Ask the patient to move his or her hand again. How has this changed his or her ability to move?

_____

_____

_____

_____

6. Turn off the unit and slowly remove the patient's hand from the unit. Carefully brush the media back into the unit and secure the sleeve.

7. What is the temperature of the unit after the treatment time?

_____

Fluidotherapy™ Application Questions

1. Was there a difference greater than 5°F between the pretreatment temperature and the posttreatment temperature of the unit? Why or why not?

_____

_____

_____

_____

2. How do the descriptions of the treatment technique sensations vary between the two patients?

_____

_____

_____

_____

3. Why do you think this is?

_____

_____

_____

_____

4. How would you describe to a patient the sensations that he or she will experience in a Fluidotherapy™ unit?

_____

_____

_____

_____

5. When would the use of a glove or bag covering the treatment area be indicated?

_____

_____

_____

_____

6. What aspect of the treatment is "lost" when a glove is worn by the patient during treatment? What is gained?

_____

_____

_____

_____

7. What are the indications for treatment with Fluidotherapy™?

_____

_____

_____

_____

Shortwave Diathermy

APPLICATION TECHNIQUES

Shortwave diathermy is a treatment modality that has been used for many years because of its ability to elevate internal tissue temperatures in relatively large treatment areas without placing anything but a towel on the surface of the skin. Because of the increased number of precautions associated with diathermy, clinicians have not always used the modality in situations in which it might be appropriate. Recent research has yielded further support for the use of diathermy as both a thermal and nonthermal treatment modality.

This exercise focuses on the thermal application techniques for diathermy and the common sensations with this application. Nonthermal application techniques would use the same principles for set-up, but there would be no reported sensation from the patient.

1. Select one of your classmates to be a patient who will have continuous thermal shortwave diathermy applied to the medial aspect of his or her knee. Inspect the area and document your observations.

_____

_____

_____

_____

2. Position the patient so that he or she will be supported and comfortable for the 15-minute treatment.

3. Drape the knee with a towel so that the towel is in contact with the skin.

4. Familiarize yourself with all of the controls of the unit. Position the treatment applicator(s), which may consist of a drum, plates, or cables. Turn the unit on.

5. Ask the patient to describe how his or her knee feels during treatment at the intervals noted and record the descriptions and your observations in the table below.

	Initially	After 3 Minutes	After 6 Minutes	After 9 Minutes	After 12 Minutes
Ask the patient to describe how his or her knee feels.					
Did the patient perspire at all during the treatment time? If yes, what did you do?					
Does the patient report any difference in sensation between the medial and lateral aspect of the knee?					

6. Turn the unit off. Remove the treatment applicator(s). Unplug the unit from the wall outlet.

7. Reassess the patient and document your observations.

_____

_____

_____

_____

Diathermy Application Questions

1. What potential advantages are there for thermal treatments with diathermy?

_____

_____

_____

_____

2. What types of patients do you think would benefit from thermal treatments with diathermy? What is your rationale for your choices?

_____

_____

_____

_____

3. What type of sensation did the diathermy produce? What type or intensity of sensation does the patient usually feel?

_____

_____

_____

_____

4. How would you explain this form of treatment to a future patient?

_____

_____

_____

_____

Cryotherapy

APPLICATION TECHNIQUES

Ice Application and Cold Water Immersion

1. Select two classmates/patients, each of whom will be having the lateral epicondyle of the humerus treated using a different form of cryotherapy. One of the patients will receive an ice massage directly to the lateral epicondyle, and the other will immerse his or her elbow in an ice bath.

2. Comfortably position both patients to support the upper extremity during treatment.

3. Wrap an ice cube in a paper towel, or use a prepared "ice pop" for the ice massage (Fig. 3-9).

4. Fill a small basin with about 3 inches of cold water and pour ice cubes or shaved ice into the water so that the entire surface of the water in the basin is covered with ice. This will serve as the ice bath (Fig. 3-10).

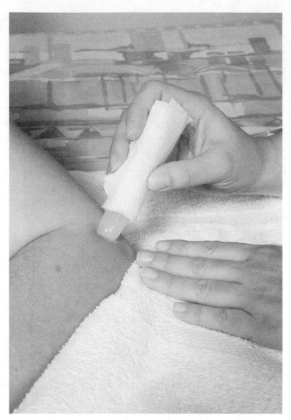

Figure 3-9 Ice massage to the lateral epicondyle with an "ice pop" wrapped in a paper towel.

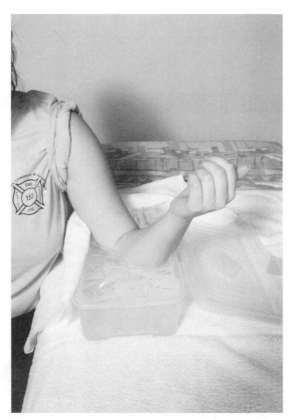

Figure 3-10 Ice bath to the lateral epicondyle. The basin is filled with ice covered with water.

5. One of the ways to help determine whether or not there is adequate circulation in a superficial area is to apply manual pressure to the area and then observe what happens. The effect is referred to as blanching, which is followed by erythema once the blood supply returns to the area after the pressure has been removed. If the circulation to an area is impaired, there will be no capillary refill or blanching effect, which would mean that cryotherapy is contraindicated for that area.

6. Check the patients for blanching over the lateral epicondyle of the humerus prior to the application of ice for this exercise.

7. Ask each patient to describe how his or her elbow feels during treatment at the intervals noted and record the descriptions and your observations in the table below.

	After 3 Minutes	After 6 Minutes	After 9 Minutes
Ice Massage			
Skin appearance			
Patient's report of how it feels			
Ice Bath			
Skin appearance			
Patient's report of how it feels			

8. With cryotherapy, a patient will feel the sensation of cold, then a burning sensation (which is normal), followed by an aching sensation, and finally numbness. The sequence is important to understand, and you should be able to explain it to patients so that they realize it is a normal series of sensations.

Ice Massage and Ice Bath Application Questions

1. Which patient experienced the greatest degree of numbness to the treated area and why?

_____

_____

_____

_____

2. Which technique was more comfortable for the patient during the treatment itself? Why?

_____

_____

_____

_____

3. In the future, how would you describe to a patient the sensations that he or she will feel during the application of ice?

_____

_____

_____

_____

4. How long did it take for each of the patients to report numbness?

Ice Massage: _____

_____

Ice Bath: _____

_____

5. How large was the area affected by the treatment in each of the patients?

Ice Massage: _____

_____

Ice Bath: _____

_____

6. Was there a relation between the size of the area affected and the time it took for numbness to occur?

_____

_____

_____

_____

7. How long did the numbness last for each of the patients?

Ice Massage: _____

_____

Ice Bath: _____

_____

8. How would you describe the appearance of the treated areas 20 minutes after the treatment?

Ice Massage: _____

_____

Ice Bath: _____

_____

9. When would you preferentially choose each of these ice modalities?

Ice Massage: _____

_____

Ice Bath: _____

_____

Commercial Ice Packs

Ice packs are available in a variety of sizes and consistencies. Several companies manufacture these packs, and they are readily available for use in the clinic and the home. Some are intended to be reusable and are therefore covered by a sturdy plastic outer layer. Other commercial cold packs may be composed of chemical compounds contained within a plastic case. Once the compounds mix, they produce a chemical reaction that results in production of a cold temperature within the pack. These packs may or may not be intended for reuse.

Regardless of the type of cold pack used, they rely on conduction as the source of thermal energy exchange. You applied commercial cold packs in several different manners in Chapter 2. All of those techniques have their place in the clinic. Whenever there are a variety of techniques for the application of something, it is the responsibility of the clinician to determine the "how and why" of the application. There may be many potential "correct" ways of doing something. What is most important is that there is a sound rationale for the choices that are made.

Refer to Chapter 2, Patient Responses to Therapeutic Interventions, for recorded patient responses to each of the commercial ice pack application techniques to answer the following questions.

1. Which patients were comfortable with the treatment itself during the ice pack application?

Directly on Skin: _____

_____

Dry Pillow Case: _____

_____

Damp Pillow Case: _____

_____

2. Which patients reported feeling numbness during the ice pack application? After how long?

Directly on Skin: _____

_____

Dry Pillow Case: _____

_____

Damp Pillow Case: _____

_____

3. Which patients responded favorably in terms of your pretreatment and treatment observations to the ice pack applications?

Directly on Skin: _____

_____

Dry Pillow Case: _____

_____

Damp Pillow Case: _____

_____

4. Were there any differences among patients in the responses that you observed? If so what were they?

Directly on Skin: _____

_____

Dry Pillow Case: _____

_____

Damp Pillow Case: _____

_____

5. Which method of application provided the patient with the least amount of conduction? The most?

Directly on Skin: _____

_____

Dry Pillow Case: _____

_____

Damp Pillow Case: _____

_____

6. Did each patient respond in some way to the respective techniques?

_____

_____

_____

_____

7. What would the rationale be for placing a layer of something, either damp or dry, between the patient and the ice pack?

_____

_____

_____

_____

8. How, if at all, did the reported sensations vary among the patients receiving the ice pack, the ice bath, and the ice massage?

Ice Pack: _____

_____

Ice Bath: _____

_____

Ice Massage: _____

_____

9. What would you inform a patient that they should feel during the application of any form of cryotherapy? (What is the sequence of sensations leading to numbness?)

First, he or she will feel:

_____

_____

After _____ minutes, they should feel:

_____

_____

After treatment, numbness which will last for about _____ minutes.

■ PATIENT SCENARIOS

Read through the patient scenarios and determine the following for each:

- Whether or not therapeutic heat would be indicated, and if so which forms
- When heat would be contraindicated
- Whether or not cryotherapy would be indicated
- When cryotherapy would be contraindicated
- If heat or cryotherapy is indicated, what your treatment goal(s) would be
- What application technique(s) you would employ (if there is more than one option, describe each)
- What precautions exist for the patient described
- What additional information, if any, you would need before applying therapeutic heat to the patient described
- What, if any, positioning considerations there are for the patient
- How you will describe to the patient what he or she should expect
- How you will assess whether or not your selection was appropriate in accomplishing your treatment goal(s)

A. John has been referred to the physical therapy department because of an injury to his left ankle. This professional hockey player, a goalie, was playing in the championship game last evening when another player collided with him on the ice. His left ankle is now edematous, particularly anterior to the lateral malleolus. He has acute tenderness in this area as well. The posterior aspect of the ankle has a large hematoma on both the medial and lateral aspects. There were no fractures noted by the physician who obtained an x-ray of the ankle last night. John's chief complaints are pain with palpation and with weight bearing, as well as an inability to don his skates due to the edema. John has no significant past medical history. He has previously encountered numerous fractures, sprains, strains, and lacerations during his career.

B. Marylou is a gymnast who has been referred to the physical therapy department for an injury that she sustained to her cervical spine when she fell from the balance beam during practice this afternoon. She complains of stiffness and pain with movements in all directions in the cervical spine. There were no fractures apparent on x-ray, and there were no abnormal neurological findings.

C. Betty is an elderly woman who was referred to the physical therapy department for treatment of her osteoarthritic hands. She has had an acute exacerbation of her arthritis after canning fresh fruits and vegetables from her garden. She lives and earns her livelihood on a farm and has rarely seen a medical professional in her lifetime. Betty has diabetes and has lost 2 toes to frostbite.

D. George is a perpetual "weekend warrior" who plays softball, soccer, and an occasional touch football game on the weekends. He has been doing this with his friends since he graduated from college in 1980. He has been referred to the physical therapy department for an injury to his right knee. He slipped on the grass during a game of "ultimate Frisbee," and he felt a sharp pain in the medial aspect of his right knee. There were no fractures identified on x-ray. He is scheduled for an MRI of the knee next week. George complains of instability, pain, and swelling in the knee. He has a history of hypertension which is being managed by medication.

E. Richard is a 55-year-old retired truck driver who has been referred to physical therapy for treatment to relieve pain and stiffness in his right knee. X-rays revealed arthritic changes in both knees. He had a medial meniscectomy in the right knee 2 years ago. His recent complaints of pain and stiffness are related to his present leisure and work activities. Richard is an avid golfer and country-and-western dancer and he works as a chauffeur.

F. Charlotte is a 50-year-old secretary who has been referred to physical therapy for treatment to relieve symptoms associated with an automobile accident that she was involved in 3 weeks ago. She is having difficulty maintaining an upright posture because of severe headaches, back pain, and intermittent paresthesias in her dominant right hand. She is a frail woman who formerly taught aerobics classes 5 nights a week. She is unable to teach at all now. There were no fractures, and she is otherwise healthy.

G. Mike is a 37-year-old carpenter who has been referred to physical therapy subsequent to a fall that took place while he was working. He fell from a second-story scaffolding while working on a house. In an attempt to break his fall, he reached for a nearby ladder and landed on a cement slab floor. His chief complaints are of pain with internal rotation, abduction, and horizontal adduction of the right shoulder. He has marked muscle guarding in the paraspinal musculature bilaterally throughout the lumbar spine. He also reinjured his left ankle, which he has sprained approximately 7 times before. As an independent contractor, he is anxious to resume work as quickly as possible to keep the project on schedule. Other than the injuries noted he has no significant medical history. His previous experiences with physical therapy were notable for unsuccessful results with ultrasound.

H. Jimmy is a 67-year-old retired factory worker who has been referred to physical therapy to help relieve chronic arthritic joint stiffness and pain in his hands. He is diabetic and has had a below-the-knee amputation on the right. He ambulates using a prosthesis and no assistive device. He is an active man who is now frustrated by his inability to work on his sailboat. He cannot tie the lines without pain, and he feels that they are insecure. This makes him dependent on others to go out sailing, which is difficult for this independent loner.

◼ DOCUMENTATION

The purpose of patient documentation is to provide an accurate record of the treatment that has been rendered. It should contain elements of the treatment technique and specific details of its application if performed in any unusual or uncustomary manner (eg, if a patient could not tolerate an ice pack unless it had two layers of cloth; if an ice bath was effective only if the temperature was 35°F). It should also provide an assessment of the patient's response to the intervention.

For the treatment to be reproduced by another clinician, or for it to be reviewed by another individual who was not there for the treatment, the documentation must include the following:

- Appearance of the skin
- Treatment modality used
  - hot packs
  - paraffin
  - Fluidotherapy™
  - diathermy
  - cryotherapy
- Area(s) treated, and what aspect of that area (e.g., medial knee; lateral knee; anterior, posterior, and lateral hip)
- How long the treatment with the modality lasted (e.g., 5 minutes, 20 minutes)
- Treatment positioning, ONLY if it was unusual (e.g., side lying, seated)
- Assessment and reassessment by the clinician with objective measures (e.g., pain scales, ROM, strength)

LAB QUESTIONS

1. Which of the therapeutic heating agents became progressively warmer during the treatment time?
2. Which of the therapeutic heating agents maintained a constant amount of heat during the treatment time?
3. Which of the therapeutic heating agents cooled off quickly after application?
4. Which of the therapeutic heating agents would be most applicable for conditions involving the hands and feet?
5. If a patient could not tolerate a prone position during the application of therapeutic heat to relieve paraspinal muscle guarding in the lower back, what alternative(s) could you provide?
6. Which of the therapeutic heat modalities would be contraindicated for a patient who has had joint replacement surgery?
7. List two treatment options for therapeutic heat application for a patient who has had joint replacement surgery.
8. What additional considerations would be necessary for positioning a patient so that the area being treated was on top of a hot pack? Is this a viable treatment option?
9. Describe the difference(s) in sensation that a patient would feel between paraffin dip and a hot pack application.
10. Describe the difference(s) in sensation that a patient would feel between hot packs and diathermy application.
11. Describe the difference(s) in sensation that a patient would feel between paraffin and Fluidotherapy™ application techniques.

Therapeutic Ultrasound

4

PURPOSE

Ultrasound is one of the most commonly used physical agent therapeutic modalities in the clinic today. There are numerous manufacturers of these devices, and there are a wide variety of parameters available. Technological advances have offered new options for treatment. It is becoming increasingly more important for clinicians to understand not only the indications, precautions, and contraindications for ultrasound but also the technology itself and how it might impact their use of ultrasound.

These lab activities start with familiarization with the devices themselves. Student/learners are guided through the identification of the parameters that are available on the devices. They are then walked through a testing procedure that will acquaint them with the beam output and some of the terminology regarding the acoustical energy beam. The lab activities are then focused around the clinical application of the previously identified parameters and the patient responses to the application of the parameters.

Student/learners are expected to be both the "patient" and the clinician so that they practice applying ultrasound as well as experience the treatment. A variety of parameters are used as well as compared and contrasted. Student/learners are expected to be able to recognize appropriate parameters for the accomplishment of a specific treatment goal as well as to be able to provide a rationale for each of their treatment decisions.

OBJECTIVES

Following the completion of this lab activity, the student/learner will be able to:

- Describe the available parameters of therapeutic ultrasound devices and the application for each of the parameters based on reported symptoms and patient status
- Describe and apply therapeutic ultrasound to accomplish a specific treatment goal, including the explanation of the treatment to the patient in terms that the patient will understand
- Use problem-solving strategies to deal with practical application challenges for ultrasound regarding:
  - patient positioning
  - parameter selection
  - device selection (based on available parameters)
- Defend the importance of performing assessment techniques before and after the application of therapeutic ultrasound to help determine its effectiveness
- Differentiate among patient responses to the application of different parameter sets of ultrasound and determine the most efficient use of ultrasound parameters based on patient responses

EQUIPMENT THAT YOU WILL NEED

variable frequency ultrasound unit (1 MHz, 3 MHz)
transducers (various sizes)
cup of water
ultrasound (acoustically-conductive) gel or lotion

towels
pillows
cellophane tape

PRECAUTIONS AND WHY

Precaution	Why?
Open wounds	Sterile saline must fill the wound for transmission of the acoustical energy.
Impaired cognitive ability	The patient must be able to communicate any uncomfortable sensation under the transducer.
Pregnancy	During the later stages of pregnancy there is no data to indicate that there would be any adverse effects as long as the treatment area does not include the abdomen, ankle,* or lower back (1 MHz).
Peripheral vascular disease	The presence of peripheral vascular disease is not a problem in itself; however, if the treatment area is involved, the patient's tissues may not be able to maintain homeostasis or respond to an increase in tissue temperature.
Advanced age	As long as the patient is alert and their sensation is intact, ultrasound should not cause any difficulties.
Previous experience with ultrasound	The patient may or may not have had a positive experience. It is important to elicit this from the patient, in addition to explaining the rationale for *this* application for *this* diagnosis.
Over joint or metal implants	Ultrasound may cause heterogenous heating within the joint if a cementing media was used. To avoid this, use 3 MHz ultrasound, which does not have sufficient depth to reach the internal aspects of joints. Metal implants tend to elevate in temperature faster than bone, but they also dissipate the heat faster, making them safe for ultrasound application.
Pain with pressure	Ultrasound involves the movement of a transducer along the surface of the skin. If this type of pressure is painful for a patient, an underwater technique with ultrasound can be employed.
Lack of sensation	Ultrasound may be administered in a thermal or a nonthermal mode. If administered in a thermal mode, the patient must be able to report pain as a potential adverse response.

*There is an acupuncture point located on the medial aspect of the ankle that may be highly active and potentially dangerous if stimulated during pregnancy.

CONTRAINDICATIONS AND WHY

Contraindications	Why?
Pregnancy	There is no physical therapy indication for application of ultrasound over a pregnant uterus, and there is no data to indicate what effect, if any, the therapeutic application of ultrasound would have on a fetus.
Abnormal growth (presumed malignant)	Thermal applications of ultrasound can potentially elevate tissue temperature, increase circulation to the area, and thus may enhance the growth.
Metastasis	Thermal applications of ultrasound can potentially elevate tissue temperature, increase circulation to the area, and thus may enhance the growth or spread malignancy to other tissues.
Lack of sensation (thermal application)	If the patient is unable to report pain, they can easily burn with thermal applications of ultrasound.
Thrombus	The application of ultrasound directly over a thrombus may cause the clot to dislodge and move to the heart, lungs, or brain.
Pacemaker	There is no indication to apply ultrasound directly over a pacemaker. The potential for interference between the pacemaker and the ultrasound device exists.
Psoriasis	Ultrasound must be applied to the skin via an acoustical media without airspace. Psoriatic skin may have too many irregularities to permit passage of the ultrasound into the patient.

LAB ACTIVITIES
Orientation to the Ultrasound Equipment

1. Select an ultrasound unit and record the information described below.

Manufacturer: _____

_____

Last Inspection Date or Manufacture Date: _____

Available Frequencies: _____

_____

Available Transducer Sizes: _____

_____

Effective Radiating Areas: _____

_____

Available Duty Cycles: _____

_____

Beam Nonuniformity Ratios: _____

_____

2. Locate each of the following components, describe them, and inspect them for wear.

Generator: _____

_____

Coaxial Cable: _____

_____

Transducer: _____

_____

Timer: _____

_____

Intensity Control: _____

_____

Duty Cycle Control: _____

_____

Testing the Transducer for Acoustical Output

Because ultrasound is usually administered without the report of any sensation from the patient, it is important to know whether or not there is any acoustical energy leaving the transducer. The water test will show visually whether or not the transducer is producing and transmitting acoustical energy. Some facilities recommend that this exercise be done weekly to ensure ultrasound output.

1. Select a transducer that is waterproof.

2. Make a ring of cellophane tape around the transducer so that you are creating a "well" that is capable of being filled with water (Figs. 4-1 and 4-2).

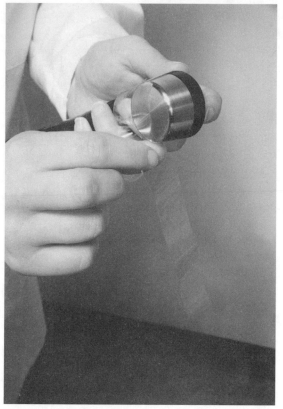

Figure 4-1 A waterproof ultrasound transducer is wrapped with cellophane tape.

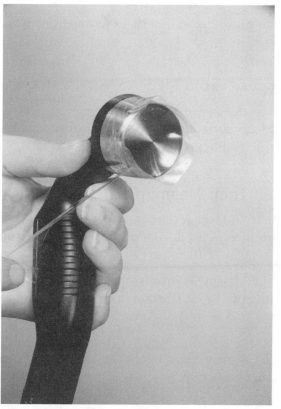

Figure 4-2 The tape wrapped around the transducer should make a complete circle capable of holding tap water.

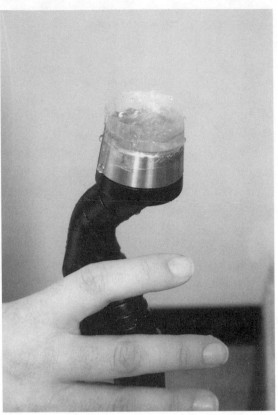

Figure 4-3 Approximately ¼ inch of tap water is added to the top of the transducer.

3. Pour some tap water into the well so that the water depth is about ¼ inch deep (Fig. 4-3).

4. Set the following parameters: 1 MHz, 1.5 W/cm^2.

5. Look at the transducer surface. If there is a disturbance in the water, then there is acoustical output from the transducer (Fig. 4-4).

Specifications and Their Meanings: ERA and BNR

1. Look down at the transducer surface from the top, and note how much of the surface of the transducer is producing disturbance in the water.

2. This is similar to looking at the effective radiating area (ERA) of the transducer. Observe the disturbance to see whether it is a high percentage or low percentage of the surface area.

3. Look at the surface of the water through the tape from the side. Gently move the water around so that you can see a cross-section of the acoustical energy leaving the transducer.

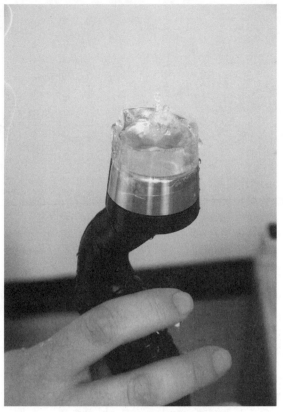

Figure 4-4 While carefully holding the transducer upright, the intensity is increased. The approximate quality of the beam is observable from both the top (effective radiating area [ERA]), and the side (beam nonuniformity ratio [BNR]).

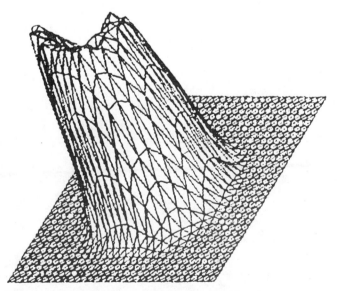

Figure 4-5 Results from an acoustical hydrophone scan depicting a uniform beam profile that also efficiently uses a high percentage of the surface area of the transducer.

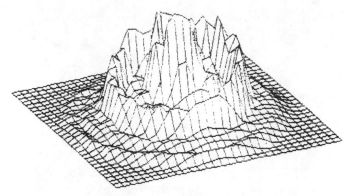

Figure 4-6 Results from an acoustical hydrophone scan depicting a beam with many peaks and valleys and a high ratio of the level of the peak output to the average output intensity.

4. This is similar to looking at the beam nonuniformity ratio (BNR) of the transducer. You are looking for uniformity to the beam. Lower BNRs are represented by fewer peaks and valleys (Fig. 4-5). Higher BNRs are represented by many peaks and valleys, and many irregularities in the beam of energy (Fig. 4-6).

◼ PROBLEM-SOLVING ACTIVITIES

Treatment Technique 1

1. Select a classmate/patient who will have his or her shoulder treated with ultrasound. Assume that the patient has a chronic supraspinatus tendinitis. The patient was evaluated by a physical therapist and the plan of care includes ultrasound to assist in decreasing joint pain, stiffness and increasing ROM, which is limited due to pain. Determine what parameters you will use and describe your rationale for their selection.

Frequency: _____

Intensity: _____

Transducer size: _____

Duty Factor: _____

Treatment Time: _____

Your Position: _____

_____

Patient Position: _____

_____

Pretreatment Assessments: _____

_____

2. Explain the treatment and anticipated effects to the patient. Use language that the patient (not a classmate) would understand.

_____

_____

_____

_____

3. Treat the patient using the parameters that you selected. Move the transducer at a speed of about 1 cm/second. What is the patient's response to the ultrasound?

_____

_____

_____

_____

4. How long after you initiated treatment with the ultrasound did sensation, if any, occur from the ultrasound?

_____

_____

5. Reassess the patient's response to treatment and document your observations.

_____

_____

_____

_____

Treatment Technique 2

1. Select a classmate/patient who will have his or her knee treated with ultrasound. Assume that the patient had an arthroscopic medial meniscectomy 2 weeks ago. The patient complains of pain at the superior medial border of the patella. ROM is limited to 0 to 50 degrees, and passive flexion produces stretching pain in the vastus medialis.

2. What area(s) will you be treating?

_____

_____

3. Determine what parameters you will use and describe your rationale for their selection.

Frequency: _____

Intensity: _____

Transducer Size: _____

Duty Factor: _____

Treatment Time: _____

Your Position: _____

_____

Patient Position: _____

_____

Pretreatment Assessments: _____

_____

4. What sensation, if any, should the patient feel during treatment?

_____

_____

_____

_____

5. If the patient does report a sensation from the ultrasound, where would you expect it to be felt (superficial or deep)?

_____

_____

_____

_____

6. What would your options be to reduce any adverse sensation?

_____

_____

_____

_____

7. Reassess the patient's response to treatment and document your observations.

_____

_____

_____

_____

Differentiating Parameter Sets for Effective Therapeutic Treatment Interventions with Ultrasound: Thermal and Nonthermal

1. Identify four classmates/patients who have palpable fibrocystic nodules in the upper trapezius that are painful to palpation. You will compare various ultrasound treatment parameter sets and report your results to your classmates and lab faculty.

2. Position and drape each patient so that he or she is comfortably supported and the upper trapezius is at rest (Fig. 4-7). All patients should be positioned identically for this exercise.

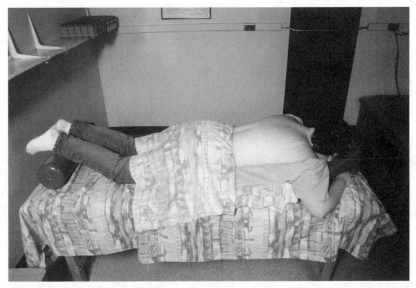

Figure 4-7 Patient positioning for uniformity and relaxation of trapezius musculature bilaterally during ultrasound application.

Patient 1	
Palpate the upper trapezius and ask the patient to rate the degree of discomfort that he or she experiences during palpation, recording it on a scale of 1–10.	

Set the following parameters: • 3 MHz • 50% DF • 0.5 W/cm^2 • For 2 minutes • Limit the treatment area to the nodule that was palpated	
What should the patient feel during the treatment?	
Re-palpate the area after treatment and record the pain rating and any change that you perceive from when you initially palpated the area.	

Patient 2 Palpate the upper trapezius and ask the patient to rate the degree of discomfort that he or she experiences during palpation, recording it on a scale of 1–10. Set the following parameters: • 3 MHz • 50% DF • 0.5 W/cm^2 • For 5 to 8 minutes depending on the transducer size (2 minutes per treatmentarea the size of the transducer) • Sonate the entire trapezius	
What should the patient feel during the treatment?	
Re-palpate the area after treatment and record the pain rating and any change that you perceive from when you initially palpated the area.	

Patient 3 Palpate the upper trapezius and ask the patient to rate the degree of discomfort that he or she experiences during palpation, recording it on a scale of 1–10.	

Set the following parameters: • 1 MHz • 100% DF • 1.5 W/cm^2 • For 5 to 8 minutes depending on the transducer size (2 minutes per treatment area the size of the transducer) • Sonate the entire trapezius	
What should the patient feel during the treatment?	
Re-palpate the area after treatment and record the pain rating and any change that you perceive from when you initially palpated the area.	

Patient 4 Palpate the upper trapezius and ask the patient to rate the degree of discomfort that he or she experiences during palpation, recording it on a scale of 1–10. Set the following parameters: • 1 MHz • 100% DF • 1.5 W/cm^2 • For 2 minutes • Sonate only the palpated nodule	
What should the patient feel during the treatment?	
Re-palpate the area after treatment and record the pain rating and any change that you perceive from when you initially palpated the area.	

Questions for Comparison

1. Which of these parameter sets produced palpable differences in the upper trapezius? Why or why not?

Patient 1 • 3 MHz • 50% DF • 0.5 W/cm^2 • For 2 minutes • Limit the treatment area to the nodule that was palpated	
Patient 2 • 3 MHz • 50% DF • 0.5 W/cm^2 • For 5 to 8 minutes depending on the transducer size (2 minutes per treatment area the size of the transducer) • Sonate the entire trapezius	
Patient 3 • 1 MHz • 100% DF • 1.5 W/cm^2 • For 5 to 8 minutes depending on the transducer size (2 minutes per treatment area the size of the transducer) • Sonate the entire trapezius	
Patient 4 • 1 MHz • 100% DF • 1.5 W/cm^2 • For 2 minutes • Sonate only the palpated nodule	

2. In what circumstances would 3 MHz be more appropriate than 1 MHz?

_____

_____

_____

_____

3. In what circumstances would pulsed ultrasound be more appropriate than continuous ultrasound?

_____

_____

_____

_____

4. In what circumstances would treating the nodule instead of the entire muscle be indicated?

_____

_____

_____

_____

■ PATIENT SCENARIOS

Read through the patient scenarios and determine the following for each:

- Which of the parameter sets for therapeutic ultrasound are indicated and provide your rationale
- What application technique you would employ
- When ultrasound would be contraindicated
- What precautions there are for the patient described
- What additional information, if any, you would need to know before applying therapeutic ultrasound to the patient described
- How you will assess whether or not your selection was appropriate in accomplishing the stated treatment goals
- How you would position the patient for treatment

A. Emma is a 55-year-old manager of a multimedia theater who has been referred to physical therapy for treatment to relieve pain and muscle guarding in her cervical spine. Her prior history includes osteoarthritis, three cervical strains, and a laminectomy and fusion of C5 and C6.

B. Cindy is a 50-year-old amateur speed trial race car driver who has been referred to physical therapy for lower back pain and muscle guarding. The pain radiates into the buttocks and down to the left popliteal space. She has a history of lower back strains due to lifting injuries while working as a roofer when she was younger. She is 5 ft tall and weighs 90 lbs. Traction relieves her radiating pain, but heat relieves her muscle guarding.

C. Phil is a 40-year-old FedEx driver who has been referred to physical therapy subsequent to intermittent pain, weakness, and cramping in his left thumb. His left hand is his dominant hand. Extension and abduction of the thumb reproduce his pain. There are no fractures, and he describes the onset of the pain as gradual. The hand is edematous with exquisite tenderness over the anatomical "snuff box."

D. Mark is a 32-year-old police officer who has been referred to physical therapy for treatment of his right forearm. He was involved in an automobile accident in which his vehicle collided head-on with another vehicle. He had multiple fractures and contusions which have now healed. His chief complaint centers on his wrist and forearm, which were fractured and pinned with a steel plate between the distal radius and ulna. He has pain with stretching of the supinators into pronation. His incision is well healed, and he has normal sensation in the upper extremity.

◼ DOCUMENTATION

For the treatment to be reproduced by another clinician, or for it to be reviewed by another individual who was not there for the treatment, the documentation must include the following information:

- Parameters of the treatment
  - frequency administered
  - duty factor
  - intensity
  - the treatment area
- The treatment time will be related to the size of the transducer that was utilized, so it is not as important to record this. However, it is still a good idea to document this information.
- It is not necessary to record the media used, unless it is something other than ultrasound gel or lotion.
- Position for treatment will be determined by the treatment goals. It needs to be recorded only if it is unusual. If stretching is taking place during the ultrasound administration, then the position and the type of stretch need to be recorded.
- Assessment and reassessment tools must be documented in the patient record.

◼ LAB QUESTIONS

1. How might knowledge of a high BNR alter the application of ultrasound?
2. How might knowledge of a low BNR alter the application of ultrasound?
3. How would knowledge of the ERA of a unit potentially benefit the clinician?
4. What tissue types absorb the greatest amount of acoustical energy?
5. Where will a patient first report a sensation from ultrasound?
6. Using terminology that a patient would understand, describe how ultrasound works, why it is not audible, and why the patient may not feel it.

7. If you were directed to use ultrasound to treat an area that was more than twice the size of the transducer and the goal was to produce heat, what would be the most appropriate action to take? Why?

8. What difference would it make if the coupling media was not acoustically conductive?

9. If a pharmacist "whipped up" a phonophoretic medication for use in the physical therapy department, what would you need to know about the mixture? And why? (Remember that whipping adds air.)

10. Outline the steps necessary for a successful treatment with phonophoresis.

Aquatics and Hydrotherapy

5

PURPOSE

This lab activity is designed to familiarize the student/learner with a wide variety of potential application techniques for water to accomplish therapeutic treatment goals. This modality is referred to as hydrotherapy.

Throughout this lab activity, student/learners are instructed to apply or experience various forms of hydrotherapy that are commonly used in the clinic today. Questions accompany each of the exercises. These questions are intended to help the student/learner learn how to incorporate the use of hydrotherapy in clinical practice for the accomplishment of clinical treatment goals.

The lab is divided into 2 parts: aquatic pools and whirlpools.

OBJECTIVES

Following the completion of this lab activity, the student/learner will be able to:

- Describe physical principles of water and how it can be therapeutically beneficial for a patient. These principles include:
  - buoyancy
  - drag
  - resistance/turbulance
- Compare a buoyant environment with a gravity environment in terms of therapeutic activities for a patient, describing which would be more challenging and which would be more supportive and why
- Describe the purpose of the components of a therapeutic whirlpool through the identification, adjustment, cleaning, and use of each of these components
- Problem-solve patient scenario difficulties in using whirlpools for patients with medical diagnoses
- Explain the advantages and disadvantages of water versus land exercise programs
- Describe the benefits of buoyancy in therapeutic exercise programs

EQUIPMENT THAT YOU WILL NEED

Whirlpools	Aquatic Pools
towels	access to a therapeutic pool
gowns	paddles (aquatic exercise devices)
whirlpool tanks (various)	stethoscope and sphygmomonometer
stethoscope and sphygmomonometer	bathing suits or T-shirts and shorts
	towels
	flotation belts

■ PRECAUTIONS AND WHY

Precaution	Why?
Healing wounds with granulation tissue	Exposure to forceful water from a turbine in a whirlpool may remove fresh granulation tissue.
Edematous extremities	Placement in a whirlpool would mean placement of the extremity in a dependent position which may increase edema.
Sensitivity or allergies to additives in water	If there are no patient sensitivities or the additives in the water, water treatment and immersion are safe; if not, the treatment is contraindicated.
Catheter	If the patient has an indwelling catheter, it is usually considered safe for the patient to be in water.
	External catheters are not considered appropriate for water submersion as they may leak or easily become dislodged.
Seizure disorder	If the patient has a seizure disorder that is treated with medication and is stable and water has not been a trigger for an event, then there is little risk. Otherwise, this type of treatment is not appropriate.
Tracheostomy	If a patient is being treated using an extremity tank, there is little risk of water entering the tracheostomy.
	If the patient is going to be placed in a Hubbard tank or aquatic environment, extreme caution should be used to prevent water from entering the tracheostomy.

■ CONTRAINDICATIONS AND WHY

Contraindication	Why?
Split-thickness skin grafts prior to 3 to 5 days	These grafts hydrate readily and may slough off when immersed in water.
Full-thickness skin grafts prior to 7 to 10 days	This type of graft takes longer before safety with water immersion can be assured. The possibility of the graft sloughing off is of great concern.

Contraindication	Why?
Full-body immersion when vital capacity is less than 1500 mL	If a patient is incapable of inflating their lungs against air pressure, they will have more difficulty inflating their lungs against the hydrostatic pressure of water, which will increase their difficulty in breathing.
IV line	This type of indwelling device would be difficult to stabilize and maintain at an adequate height to allow the administration of medication in an Whirlpool treatment might be a viable option.
Colostomy	This type of opening cannot be adequately sealed to prevent leakage into the pool or leakage of water back into the patient. Water immersion in an aquatic environment must not include a colostomy.
Incontinent	Patients who are incontinent should not enter an aquatic environment, where voiding will contaminate the water for others.
Fever	Patients with an active infection who are febrile should not be placed in an aquatic environment in which the water temperature might further increase their core temperature.

■ LAB ACTIVITIES

Orientation to Therapeutic Aquatic Pools

Experiencing Buoyancy and Resistance in Water

Buoyancy is a force present underwater that is not present on land. It acts in opposition to the force of gravity. For this reason, virtually everything that is limited due to gravity on land can be performed more easily with the support of buoyancy.

Land	Aquatic
Against gravity	Buoyancy assisted
With gravity	Buoyancy resisted
Gravity eliminated	Buoyancy supported

To facilitate learning about these differences, it will be necessary for you to have access to a therapeutic pool with varied depth from about 2 ft to more than 6 ft. Because you will be exercising in the pool, as would your patients, the pool temperature is an important consideration.

Therapeutic exercise	94°F ($\pm$2°F)
Therapeutic heat	104°F (*not appropriate for a pool!*)

1. Have a classmate record your vital signs and a few other pieces of data before and after you enter the water.

	Before Therapy	After Therapy
Heart rate		
Blood pressure		
Respiration		
Pool temperature		
Time		

2. You will be in a therapeutic pool for the following activities. It is suggested that you appoint a classmate to read and record your responses from the activities while you are in the water.

3. Walk in water of various depths and describe the difference each makes in your ease of movement.

   Knee Deep: _____

   _____

   Waist Deep: _____

   _____

   Shoulder Deep: _____

   _____

4. In shoulder-depth water, perform the following activities and describe what happens and why.

   Walk Forward: _____

   _____

   Stop Quickly: _____

   _____

   Try to Run: _____

   _____

5. Stand in shoulder-depth water and slowly horizontally abduct your right shoulder, stopping at 45 degrees.

   • Does your arm have a tendency to move or stop in this position?

   _____

   _____

   • Would this be a gravity-assisted position on land?

   _____

   _____

   • How would you describe the position in the water (buoyancy resisted or buoyancy assisted)?

   _____

   _____

6. What could you do to increase the amount of resistance to movement that you encounter in the water? Try it. Does it work?

   _____

   _____

   _____

   _____

7. If a patient tried your technique to increase the resistance, would there be any additional considerations? If yes, what would they be?

   _____

   _____

   _____

   _____

8. What happens when you push your hands down to your sides from the surface of the water with your forearms pronated?

   _____

   _____

   _____

   _____

- What happens when you repeat this with your forearms in a neutral position? Why?

_____

_____

_____

_____

9. Float in the water with your shoulders abducted to 90 degrees. Once you are floating, what happens when you extend your hip?

_____

_____

_____

_____

- For what exercise or motion would this position provide buoyancy assistance and resistance?

_____

_____

_____

_____

10. Apply a deep water belt securely around your waist before entering the deep end of the pool. If you have a tendency to sink, you may need to apply more than one belt. Move into the deep end of the pool where the depth of the water exceeds your height. "Walk" in the deep water so that your body remains vertical. Perform the following activities and record your observations below.

	What Happened?	How Much Effort Was Required?	How Much Weight Bearing Took Place?
Walk forward			
Walk backward			

	What Happened?	How Much Effort Was Required?	How Much Weight Bearing Took Place?
Ski			
Scissor your legs			
Bring your knees up to your chest			
Lower your knees			

11. Come out of the pool, and record the same data as when you entered the pool in the table in question 1. Also record the following:

   • How long were you in the pool?

   _____

   _____

   • How, if at all, did your vital signs change? Why or why not?

   _____

   _____

   _____

   _____

12. Based on any changes in your vital signs, what impact would similar changes have on patients involved in aquatic pool programs?

   _____

   _____

   _____

   _____

Whirlpools

Orientation to the Equipment

1. Identify and name each piece of hydrotherapy equipment in Figures 5-1 through 5-3.

   • Find and label the turbine on each of the whirlpools.
   • Find and label the aeration adjustment on the turbines and locate the breather opening(s).

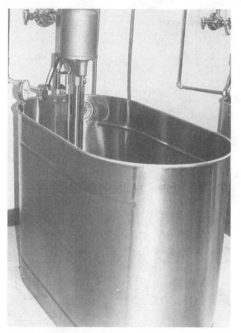

Figure 5-1 Common style of stainless steel whirlpool.

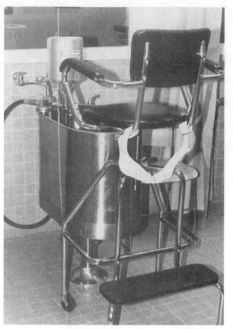

Figure 5-2 Common style of stainless steel whirlpool.

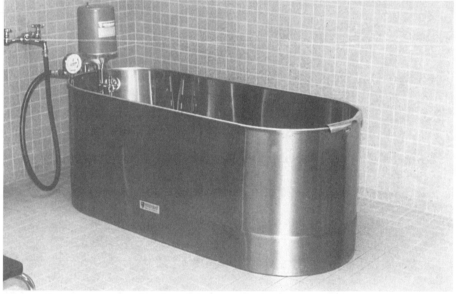

Figure 5-3 Common style of stainless steel whirlpool.

2. Record your observations of the various kinds of tanks in the table below.

	High Boy	**Low Boy**	**Extremity Tank**
How many gallons of water does this tank hold?			
What areas of the body could be treated in this tank?			

	High Boy	Low Boy	Extremity Tank
Fill and empty the tanks, recording the time to fill and your technique for filling the tank to maintain the water at 104°F.*			

*While the tank is full, perform the activities listed in Problem-Solving Activities, below.

■ PROBLEM-SOLVING ACTIVITIES

Transfers and Patient Positioning With Whirlpools

Low Boy

1. Transfer a patient into the low boy from a wheelchair. He or she is non–weight bearing (NWB) on the left lower extremity (LLE). The patient has no significant past medical history (PMH).

   • What planning is required for you to accomplish this task safely?

   _____

   _____

   _____

   _____

   • What else do you need to know about the patient before you transfer him or her into the tank?

   _____

   _____

   _____

   _____

   • Of what significance is the water level in the tank prior to transferring the patient into the tank?

   _____

   _____

   _____

   _____

- What transfer aids, if any, did or would you use?

  _____

  _____

  _____

  _____

- Describe the sequence for the transfer and any difficulties that you may have had, outlining how you would approach it the next time.

  _____

  _____

  _____

2. Adjust the patient's position so that he or she is long-sitting in the low boy. Support the patient's back and arms so that no excess pressure is exerted on them. (A towel roll may be used to cushion the extremities from the edges of the tank.)

3. Turn on the turbine and adjust it so that the turbulence is directed at a 45-degree angle to the left side of the tank.

   - What sensation does the patient report?

     _____

     _____

     _____

   - Where does the patient feel the agitation?

     _____

     _____

     _____

- Decrease the amount of air that flows into the turbine. How does this change the sensation that the patient has reported?

  _____

  _____

  _____

  _____

- Increase the amount of air flow to maximum. How does this change the sensation reported by the patient, if at all?

  _____

  _____

  _____

  _____

4. Adjust the turbine so that it is pointing directly at the patient.

   - What is the patient's response to the adjustment?

     _____

     _____

     _____

     _____

   - After 5 minutes of submersion and adjustments to the turbine air flow, recheck the water temperature. Has it changed? If yes, why?

     _____

     _____

     _____

     _____

5. Prepare your patient to be transferred out of the tank and back into the wheelchair. List the steps that you need to perform.

   _____

   _____

   _____

   _____

6. Repeat the transfer in and out of the low boy until you are comfortable with what you will need to consider to ensure patient and personal safety.

Extremity Tank

1. Position your patient to have his or her right foot treated in the extremity tank. What considerations do you need to make?

_____

_____

_____

_____

2. Adjust the turbine to perform nonspecific débridement to a fragile calcaneal ulcer. What considerations do you need to make, and how would you adjust the turbine?

_____

_____

_____

_____

3. What would change if the patient were being treated for an acute ankle sprain?

_____

_____

_____

_____

4. Describe some of the problems you encountered and how you addressed them.

_____

_____

_____

_____

Patient Transfers in the Hubbard Tank

1. Demonstrate the use of the Hubbard tank and its lift by transferring one of your classmates into the tank. As appropriate for the use of the Hubbard tank itself and for the lift, describe the following:

Patient Instructions: _____

_____

Indications: _____

_____

Contraindications: _____

_____

Precautions: _____

_____

Cleaning the Whirlpool Tanks

1. Empty and clean each of the tanks that were used and describe the procedure.

_____

_____

_____

_____

2. Where did you find the information for cleaning the tanks?

_____

_____

_____

_____

3. What is the procedure for cleaning the turbines?

_____

_____

_____

_____

4. Why do the turbines need to run while cleaning?

_____

_____

_____

_____

▰ PATIENT SCENARIOS

Read through the patient scenarios and determine the following for each:

- Whether hydrotherapy is indicated
- What equipment you would use
- The optimal water temperature
- Whether agitation should be used
- The potential benefits of hydrotherapy

A. Hazel is a slender 80-year-old woman with a left (L) calcaneal decubitus ulcer. She has a past medical history (PMH) of diabetes.

B. John is a 25-year-old man status post (s/p) open reduction and internal fixation (ORIF) of the right (R) ankle and spasm of the right calf musculature. His incision is well healed, and he is partial weight bearing (PWB) on the R leg with crutches. His ROM in dorsiflexion and plantarflexion are limited.

C. Janet is a 60-year-old woman s/p R long-leg cast removal. She lives alone in a first-floor condominium and has been ambulating non–weight bearing (NWB) on the R leg with a walker. She has good strength throughout her upper extremities (UEs) and lower extremities (LEs). She is anxious to resume her schedule, which included aerobics and bicycling.

D. Mike is a 35-year-old man who experienced a traumatic amputation of his left upper extremity (LUE) above the elbow. The injury occurred 8 weeks ago. He is anxious to resume working. His amputation scar is well healed, and he will be fitted with a prosthesis as soon as the residual limb is toughened up. His UE strength is poor, and he fatigues easily since the injury. He has inquired about a possible home therapy program.

E. Marty is a 55-year-old woman who is 8 weeks s/p transtibial amputation of the RLE secondary to insensate ulcerations as a result of diabetes. She is anxious to be fitted for a prosthesis and to begin ambulation. Her incision is well healed, and she has no other significant PMH.

F. Mary is a 68-year-old obese woman with severe osteoporosis of the hip bilaterally. She was referred to the physical therapy department after a fall that resulted in a compound fracture of the L femur. The fracture has healed. Goals include increasing strength and promoting weight bearing to prevent further bone loss.

G. Bill is a 45-year-old man s/p 8 weeks lumbar laminectomy who has bilateral muscle guarding of the paraspinal musculature. He is working as an architect and is limited in all spinal movement because of this muscle guarding. He formerly was very active as a triathlete. He needs mobility and aerobic exercises that will allow the paraspinal muscles to relax.

H. Brian is a 22-year-old man with an acute sprain (3 days ago) of the anterior talofibular ligament of the right ankle. His ankle is edematous but pain-free. His ankle ROM is limited in all directions by muscle guarding. He is anxious to return to work as a mail carrier.

I. Sharon is a 68-year-old woman s/p R radical mastectomy with decreased shoulder ROM in all directions. Her incisions are well healed, and she is anxious to resume as much activity as possible. She had been an aerobics instructor for a senior citizen center.

J. Jack is a 45-year-old man s/p 4 weeks arthroscopic meniscectomy of the L knee 4 weeks ago. His incision is well healed, and he is now fully weight bearing (FWB) on the L leg. He complains of weakness and that his knee "gives out" when he descends stairs.

■ DOCUMENTATION

The purpose of documentation is to provide an accurate record of the treatment that has been rendered. It should contain elements of the treatment technique and specific details of its application if performed in any unusual or uncustomary manner. It should also provide an assessment of the patient's response to the treatment intervention.

For the treatment to be reproduced by another clinician, or for it to be reviewed by another individual who was not there for the treatment, the documentation must include the following:

- Type of hydrotherapy intervention used (aquatic pool or whirlpool)
- For whirlpools, documentation should also include:
  - temperature of the water
  - whether agitation was used
  - whether any additives were used in the water
- For aquatic pools, documentation should also include:
  - temperature of the water
  - depth of immersion
  - treatment time
  - any special equipment
- Any significant changes in the vital signs of the patient should also be recorded, along with an assessment and plan based on these changes.

■ LAB QUESTIONS

1. Approximately how long should you allow for the preparation of a whirlpool?
2. What additional considerations are there for positioning and body mechanics with high-boy and low-boy whirlpools?
3. Describe the benefits of nonspecific débridement.
4. Describe the potential adverse effect that a turbine can cause to a healing ulcer and how the harm could be prevented.
5. Your patient has been diagnosed with a spinal cord injury that is now stable at T4. What potential reasons are there to have the patient participate in an aquatic pool program?
6. What additional benefits are derived from deep-water activities in an aquatic pool that are not possible through land exercises?
7. Other than ROM in a buoyancy-assisted environment, what are the benefits of aquatic therapy for postmastectomy patients?
8. Describe how flotation devices can be used to increase the level of resistance for an exercise program.

Soft Tissue Treatment Techniques: Traction

6

PURPOSE

This lab activity is designed to demonstrate the principles of therapeutic traction that are currently practiced in clinical environments. Student/learners will become familiar with the treatment goals, positioning, apparatus, and techniques that are commonly employed. Student/learners will administer and receive various forms of traction and learn the importance of proper positioning for both the patient and the device or individual applying the traction. This lab activity also covers what to document and how important appropriate patient instruction is to treatment success.

OBJECTIVES

Following the completion of this lab activity, the student/learner will be able to:

- Discuss the importance of appropriate patient positioning techniques for the application of traction by describing the line of pull and the impact of gravity
- Discuss current theories behind the application of cervical and lumbar traction
- Demonstrate techniques to decrease the stresses on postural muscles so that a traction force may be successfully applied to the cervical musculature
- Identify the controls on mechanical traction equipment devices and describe their functions for potential patient application
- Demonstrate the proper application of supports, belts, and straps to accomplish mechanical traction
- Demonstrate problem-solving techniques for patient stabilization during the application of manual traction
- Describe what various forms or traction feel like when applied and relate this experience to a patient

EQUIPMENT THAT YOU WILL NEED

mechanical traction unit (with instruction manual)
belts and straps for traction unit
cervical traction head halter
treatment table
Saunders™ cervical traction appliance

goniometer
foot stool
pillows
towels

Mock-up Cervical Traction Model Set-up (Optional)

empty plastic gallon milk bottle
level (small plastic bubble level)
cloth straps (about 3 yd)

string plum bob
protractor
adhesive tape

PRECAUTIONS AND WHY

Precaution	Why?
Joint hypermobility (spinal)	The pull that is applied with traction may exacerbate joint instability unless it is carefully monitored.
Pregnancy	The lumbar belts that must be applied to administer mechanical lumbar traction may be inappropriate depending on the delivery date.
Acute inflammation (spinal)	After an acute injury, there may be muscle guarding, which would impair the patient's ability to relax during the application of traction. This may lead to minor muscle tearing, which could increase the patient's symptoms.
Claustrophobia	Patients who have difficulty with confinement or closed spaces may experience increased muscle guarding during the application of mechanical traction.
Temporomandibular joint dysfunction	The cervical halter used for these patients must be one that does not apply any pressure on the mandible or mechanical cervical traction may exacerbate their TMJ dysfunction.

CONTRAINDICATIONS AND WHY

Contraindication	Why?
Spinal infection	The possibility exists that infection could be spread through the use of spinal traction.
Rheumatoid arthritis	The integrity of the joint is compromised by the disease process. The addition of a traction force may further increase joint instability without providing any relief for the patient.
Osteoporosis	The application of mechanical traction may cause fragile bone to fracture either through the pull of the traction or the tightness of the straps.
Spinal cancer	Increasing circulation to the spinal structures through the use of spinal traction may encourage the spread of the malignancy via seeding.
Cardiac or respiratory insufficiency or recent ophthalmic surgery	Inversion traction is the only form of traction contra-indicated in these patients because it increases internal pressure.
Spinal cord pressure secondary to central disk herniation	Patients with major involvement of the intervertebral disc, including central disc herniation, will receive no sustained benefit from externally applied traction.

Special Considerations for the Application of Traction

- Traction must be terminated and the patient must be re-evaluated if symptoms worsen during its application.
- Patients must be given a shut-off button (if available) or call button to use in case of emergency.

Orientation to Patient Positioning for Traction

Traction can be defined as a process of pulling or drawing apart. This process involves pulling or separating joint surfaces. Traction can be applied manually or mechanically. Regardless of the technique, patient positioning to accomplish the goal is an integral part of the process. Without proper positioning, the line of pull may not be capable of accomplishing the separation desired.

Supine

1. Have one of your classmates lie supine on a plinth without any pillows. Position them so that there is a straight line along midline bisecting their right and left sides.

   - What was/were your point(s) of reference to determine that they were "straight"?

     1- The head was facing straight up in neutral position
     2- Shoulders were even
     3- Trunk in proper alignment c̄ midline
     4- Hip is even
     5- Arm length on equal at the sides of their trunk
     6- Legs are aligned straight c̄ the head & Trunk. Legs are at an even lengthy c̄ each.

   - Is the patient comfortable in this position?

     OK

   - What is the position of the lumbar spine? (Is there a lordosis?)

     There is lordosis when the hip & knees are extended
     There is not lordosis when hip & knees are flexed.
     (cervical lordosis)

   - What is the position of the cervical spine?

     Neutral Position. The head facing up (forward) c̄ no flexion
     No Flexion, rotation or lat bending of the
     head & neck. The ears align c̄ AC joint.

2. Position your classmate so that they have a flat lumbar lordosis and a neutral cervical lordosis (Figs. 6-1 and 6-2).

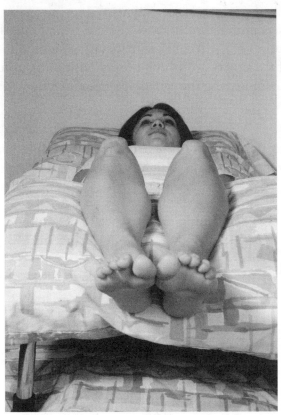

Figure 6-1 Patient positioned supine with midline in proper alignment with all bony landmarks.

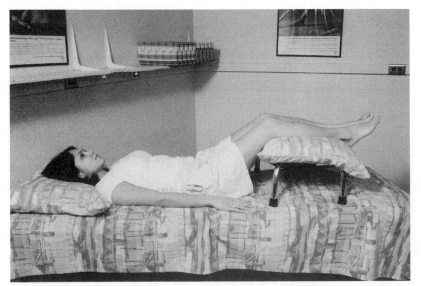

Figure 6-2 Patient positioned in supine with a flat lumbar lordosis as viewed from the side.

- Describe what you had to do to accomplish this.

  Placed a pillow under the head and had had the pt position their head in a neutral position facing up.

- Is the patient comfortable in this position?

  Yes

- Is the patient still "straight" with a bisecting midline?

  Yes

- How long does it take to position the patient so that he or she has both a flat lordosis and a neutral cervical spine?

  About a minute

3. Grasp the humerus of your classmate, superior to the distal epiphysis, so that you can apply gross distraction/traction to the right upper extremity.

- What happens to the alignment of the patient?

  The pts (R) UE shifts down. The spine will lateral bend to the right. Shoulders are uneven lateral.

- How much traction force did it take for the alignment to shift (a lot, some, hardly any)?

  It takes hardly any traction force to shift the alignment

4. Have another classmate stabilize the acromion process of the scapula and trunk while you distract the humerus.

- What happens to the alignment of the patient?

  The alignment of the pt doesn't have a significant change

- How much traction force did it take for the alignment to shift (a lot, some, hardly any)?

  It take a lot of traction force to shift the alignment

- What purpose would stabilization serve when applying traction?

  The purpose of stabilization during Traction is to help maintain alignment; reduce frictions; help with maximum pull & distraction of vertebrals.

Sitting

1. Have one of your classmates sit in a chair that has a straight back (armrests optional). He or she should be positioned so that the feet are flat and firmly touching the floor in an erect posture with a straight line running from the external auditory meatus of the ear through the acromion process, the spine, and the greater trochanter.

   - Describe what you had to do to accomplish this.

     Placed a towel roll behind the lumbar section of the back

   - What tools did you use to assess the patient's position?

     Plumb line, or yard stick

   - Is the patient comfortable in this position?

     Yes

   - How long did it take to accomplish this position?

     Minute

- While you were recording your answers, did the patient shift position? If yes, how?

  Yes

- If your goal was to relieve the pressure of the head on the cervical spine created by gravity, where would the "pull" need to come from?

  To relieve the pressure of the head on the cervical spine, the "pull" needs to come from the opposite direction of the force of gravity c̄ the neck in 30° of flexion.

- How would you stabilize the rest of the body?

  The back support of the chair or the whole chair would need to be tild back. The pts body weight and gravity would stabilize the rest of the body.

2. Select one of the cervical head halters and inspect it. Determine which is the mandibular strap and which is the occipital strap. With the patient seated, place the halter on him or her. There should be some kind of adjustment that can be made between the mandibular and occipital straps. Adjust the straps with a hand on each side of the head. Gently pull upward to take up the slack in the straps; do not try to relieve the weight of the head.

- If your goal was to relieve the weight of the head, what direction or angle should the traction pull toward?

  To relieve the weight of the head the angle of pull should be 25° – 35° / upright – vertical

- Why is it important not to have the pull come from the mandible?

It is important not to have the pull come from the mandible because it can create and aggravate Temporomandibular Joint Problems.

- How difficult is it to adjust the line of pull to accomplish an occipital pull? What do you need to do?

In a sitting position, it would be slightly difficult depending the chair. One must need a reclining chair to accomplish an occipital pull.

3. What would the rationale be for an occipital pull? What would be accomplished?

There are no mandibular strap and the pull is exclusively the occiput.

4. What is/are the treatment goal(s) of cervical traction? C tx
① Reduction of radicular sign & symptons associated w/ condition such as disc protrusion, lateral stenosis, degenerative disc disease, and subluxations (spondylolisthesis)
② Reduction of joint pain via neurophysiologic pathways (gatting mechanism)
③ Increase ROM via distraction / mobilization of joint surfaces.

5. How would you know if a patient was responding favorably to the application of cervical traction? How would his or her symptoms change?

The PTA must as how the pt feels before and after the treatment. There may have decreased pain, decrease numbness, & increase in ROM.

Mock Cervical Traction Set-up (Optional)

1. Fill an empty gallon milk container with water and re-cap it, securing the cap with a ring of adhesive tape. The bottle will represent the head for this exercise. The handle of the milk bottle represents the posterior upper cervical spine as it comes from the base of the occiput. The cap of the bottle is inferior to the chin.

2. Place a ring of adhesive tape around the base of the occiput, and around the entire head (bottle) so that it bisects the head just below the nose. The line of tape should be perpendicular to the seam on the bottle (Fig. 6-3).

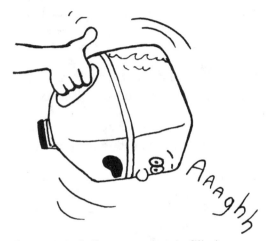

Figure 6-3 Gallon water bottle filled, capped off, and marked with tape to indicate the position of horizontal midline and the occiput.

3. Place another line of tape on the anterior seam on the bottle. This will be an additional reference point for positioning.

4. Attach the level to one side of the bottle so that it is parallel to the seam and perpendicular to the occipital tape ring.

5. You will note that handling the bottle full of water is not easy. The weight of the gallon container is approximately 8 lb, which actually is less than the weight of the human head.

6. You will also note that resting the bottle on the table so that the seam is facing up and is aligned is not easy either. The human head is much the same. The patient will have a tendency to turn their head to one side to rest as it does not easily balance in neutral (Fig. 6-4).

7. Take the cloth tape and make a cervical halter similar to the prefabricated one that you previously inspected and worked with. Start by making a loop that is about 24 inches long when folded. Make two tape rings for this loop; they will represent the metal D-rings that you held on the prefabricated cervical halter (Fig. 6-5).

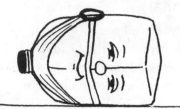

Figure 6-4 Gallon water bottle lying on its side and wearing a cervical head halter.

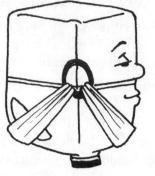

Figure 6-5 Gallon water bottle in erect posture and wearing a cervical head halter.

8. Build an occipital strap and a mandibular strap with tape so that the bony prominences of the head ("bottle") will have a place to catch onto.

9. Apply your cervical halter to the bottle. Determine what angle the line of pull should be to relieve the weight of the head while maintaining the level in a fixed position (Fig. 6-6).

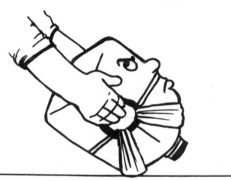

Figure 6-6 Manual adjustment of the line of pull on the halter to attempt to pull from the occiput.

Manual Cervical Traction Demonstration

1. Ask one of your lab instructors to demonstrate manual cervical traction with the patient in a seated and a supine position.

   • Which position appeared "easier" for the clinician? Why?

   Sitting appears "easier" for the clinician b/c body mechanisms is easier to control and less gravity is acting on the spine

- Which position appeared more comfortable for the patient? Why?

Supine appears more comfortable for the pt. There is less gravitational pull. The body is stabilized easier. The head is more relaxed.

2. Cervical traction is usually applied in the supine position. Why do you think this is?

Provides improved muscle relaxation, vertebral separation and easier conter traction.

3. Ask one of the lab instructors to set up the Saunders™ cervical traction appliance by attaching it to a mechanical traction unit (Fig. 6-7).

- Before a patient is positioned on the plinth, what can you predict about the position in which the appliance will place the cervical spine?

The cervical spine will be in a supinated and flexed postion

- Inspect the appliance. What is the purpose of the small sled on which the occiput rests?

Reduce friction, support the head, and the pull the vertebrae

- Inspect the straps and supports for the appliance. What is the purpose of the temporal/frontal strap?

Stablize the head in place

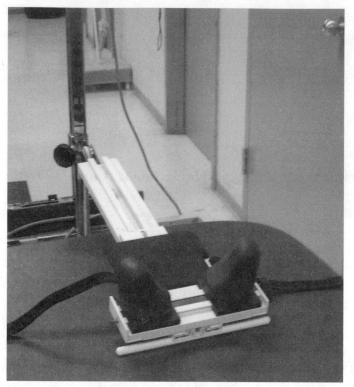

Figure 6-7 Saunders™ cervical traction appliance attached to a mechanical traction unit.

- How is the mandible treated with this appliance? (Is there any support for it or pull on it?)

  There is not support or pull on the mandible

4. If you were to give your seated cervical traction patient a magazine to pass the time while they were in traction, what would happen to his or her positioning?

   the head and neck may shift into a different position

5. If you were to instruct a supine patient to "just get up" after a traction force had been applied and released, what would happen to the intra-disc pressure?

Intra disc press would decrease ✓

6. Why would the position of the patient prior to the application of a traction force make a difference?

The position of the pt may change their pain (increase or decrease the pain)

7. How much force would it take to overcome the weight of the head?

Sitting: 25 - 45 lbs

Supine: 25 - 45 lbs

Supine with Cervical Appliance: 25 - 45 lbs

8. What happened to the pressure on the mandible when you tried to adjust the angle of pull to the occiput on the bottle?

The pressure on the mandible increases as the angle becomes more vertical

9. The cervical spine has 2 individual curves. Of what significance are they when applying cervical traction?

The 2 individual curves has different angle of pull. Segments below C2, the cervical spine in 20 to 30 of flexion. If the atlantoaxial segment is Treated allow the normal lordosis To remain and 0 degrees of flex to treat the pt.

10. What muscles maintain the normal cervical curves?

Rectus capitis posterior major, rectus capitis posterior minor, obliquus capitis superior, obliquus capitis inferior

11. Which muscles tend to guard following a cervical strain? What impact, if any, would guarding in these muscles have on the curves of the cervical spine?

Splenius capitis, splenius cervicis, sternomastoid, levator scapuli, scalenes

Lumbar Traction Demonstration

1. Observe while one of your lab instructors demonstrates manual lumbar traction with the patient in supine position with hips and knees flexed.

   • What problems do you see for the clinician in maintaining this level of traction?

   Therapist may become fatigued and not be able to provide a constant significant traction face

   • Which position appeared to be more comfortable for the patient? Why?

   Supine with the hips & knees slightly flexed, the back is supported, but the legs are not sticking up in the air

   • How much traction force was the clinician able to apply manually, and how reproducible would this be from clinician to clinician? Why?

   Traction face depends on the strength of the therapist. It would be difficult for another therapist to apply the same amount of face because the amount of face is subjective

2. Lumbar traction is usually applied with mechanical devices. Why do you think this is?

The same amount of force can be applied with each pull, mechanical traction may be tiring for the therapist and difficult to maintain

3. Observe while one of the lab instructors sets up the thoracic and lumbar traction belts and straps and attaches them to the mechanical traction unit.

   - Before a patient is positioned on the plinth, what can you predict about the position in which the appliance will place the lumbar spine?

     Lordotic

   - Inspect the set-up. Why were straps applied to the thoracic and lumbar areas?

     The straps on the lumbar harness allow you to provide traction, the straps on the thoracic harness provide countertraction and keep pt from sliding on table

   - Why was padding added to the straps?

     The straps may be uncomfortable to the pt, especially if the pt is thin

   - Why were the hips flexed? What did this do to the lumbar spine?

     The hips flexed creates flexion of lumbar spine / posterior wedging of the disc, increased foraminal space, and decreased WB forces on facets.

4. If you were to instruct a supine patient to "just get up" after a traction force had been applied and released, what would happen to the intra-disc pressure?

The intra disc pressure could increase

5. Why would the position of the patient prior to the application of a traction force make a difference?

The position of the pt determines the angle of pull & whether the pull is lordotic or kyphotic

6. How much force would it take to overcome the weight of the lower half of the body in the supine position?

A minimum of 1/4 the pt's body weight and no more than 50% — 60% depending on pt tolerance and results of tx.

• If you are using a traction table that splits, does this make a difference? If so how?

Yes A split traction table reduces the friction face to almost 0.

7. What happens to the pressure on the lumbar spine when the angle of pull is adjusted?

Adjusting the angle of pull can increase or increase the pressure depending on the angle

8. Which muscles tend to guard following a lumbar strain? What impact, if any, would guarding in these muscles have on the curves of the lumbar spine?

   Quatratus Lumborum, Rectus abdominis, Ext & Internal Obliques, Rotatores, Multifidis, Erector spinae

9. Apply lumbar traction to a classmate, and have a classmate apply lumbar traction to you. Use the poundage suggested by your lab instructor. Record your observations regarding how the traction felt.

   Your Observations: *Straps were uncomfortable it seemed harder to breath*

   Classmate's Observations: *He hardly felt any pull at 1/4 his body wt.*

10. What instructions did your lab instructor provide to the "sample patient" that you would use in the future? Why?

    Instructions on kill switch - Safety same instructions about getting up from table. Safest way to get up.

11. It is important to ask a patient whether or not he or she needs to use the restroom before the application of lumbar traction. Why do you believe that this would be an important consideration?

    It takes time & effort to get the pt into the harnesses & hooked up to traction machine. You don't want to have to unhook anything unless it's absolutely necessary

PATIENT SCENARIOS

A. If you were instructed to apply cervical traction for the reduction of cervical muscle pain and guarding in a patient who had unilateral guarding of the upper trapezius on the right, what, if anything, about the treatment set-up would change? Why?

B. Matt is a 45-year-old construction worker who injured his back while installing a steel grate to cover a drainage basin. He has no other significant past medical history. His back and leg pain occurred after he let go of the grate, when he attempted to straighten up. He now has radicular symptoms in the left leg from the buttocks down to the lateral malleolus. His strength and sensation are normal. His primary complaint is that of pain down the back of his leg. He is anxious to return to work. Would traction of some form be indicated? If yes, how? If not, why? What additional considerations might there be for this patient?

C. Sue was referred to therapy for evaluation and treatment of her cervical pain symptoms. Her physician recommended that traction be considered along with other palliative modalities to relieve her discomfort and improve her mobility. This physician is eager to discuss this patient with the evaluating therapist to discuss treatment options. Sue was injured in an automobile accident in which her car was struck from behind. She has bilateral guarding in all cervical muscles. She recently underwent a mandibular reduction to correct horizontal alignment of her incisors. What additional considerations are there for this patient? Would traction be contraindicated? Why or why not?

D. Will has been referred to therapy by his family physician for lumbar traction to relieve questionable lumbar radiculopathies that appear to be transient. Will injured his back while working, and he has not returned to work yet. He works as an architect. His complaints of pain and numbness vary. Some days, the paresthesia is located in the right foot and other days it is in the left foot. Traction was suggested to determine if centralization of the pain was possible. There were no signs of fracture. After examination and discussion, traction was initiated to determine whether or not it would provide any sustained benefit.

E. One day after receiving his first treatment with traction, Will returns to the clinic for another treatment. He states that his symptoms subsided following the traction. Today, his paresthesia is behind his left knee, but he also complains of pain in the right buttocks. When setting up the lumbar belts, you ask him whether he needs to use the restroom before receiving traction. Will declines and states that he has not been able to urinate for about the last 12 hours. What course of action should you take? Why?

■ DOCUMENTATION

As with other modalities, it is important to document the parameters administered to a patient. When using traction, this is particularly important. The following parameters must be documented:

- Patient position (e.g., supine, knees flexed or extended, prone, sitting)
- Type of traction
  - mechanical
  - intermittent
  - sustained
  - manual
- Amount of force in pounds

- Duration
  - hold time
  - rest time
- Attachments
  - Saunders™ cervical traction
  - cervical halter
  - over-the-door home unit
- Total treatment time

It is also important to document the patient's initial complaint before traction and his or her response to the traction. Traction is commonly applied to relieve radicular symptoms. Record whether the goal was accomplished subsequent to the application of traction. Sometimes a patient will report a decrease in symptoms during traction but a return of the symptoms once the traction force is released. This must also be documented.

LAB QUESTIONS

1. Describe how your body mechanics might change if you performed manual cervical traction while a patient was seated in a chair and while lying supine.
2. If cervical and lumbar traction are performed to relieve radiculopathies, what is the goal of appendicular manual traction?
3. Of what significance is hand placement of the individual who is stabilizing the patient during a manual traction treatment?

Soft Tissue Management Techniques: Edema Management

7

PURPOSE

This lab activity focuses on therapeutic techniques for the management of edema. Clearly, there are multiple causes for edema, and it is a complex problem for both the patient and the clinician to deal with. Student/learners will practice assessment techniques for edema, because without accurate measurement of the edema it is impossible to determine whether or not the technique used proved effective. Part of the lab activity also focuses on treatment techniques with the use of intermittent compression devices.

OBJECTIVES

Following the completion of this lab activity, the student/learner will be able to:

- Demonstrate edema assessment techniques for the upper and lower extremity, including use of a volumeter and tape measure
- Demonstrate patient positioning for, clinical application of, and removal of an intermittent compression device for edema reduction in the upper and lower extremity
- Demonstrate the monitoring of pedal, popliteal, and radial pulses on classmates and indicate the clinical relevance of these for patient populations with edematous extremities

EQUIPMENT THAT YOU WILL NEED

vinyl tape measure
goniometer
upper extremity volumeter
foot volumeter
catch basin for water
large graduated cylinder
stethoscope

thermometer
marking pen
sphygmomanometer
intermittent compression device
upper and lower extremity appliances
   for compression device
disposable stockinet

PRECAUTIONS AND WHY

Precaution	Why?
Diuretics	Patients taking diuretics may need more frequent breaks for voiding.
Decreased cognitive ability	If the patient is capable of communicating discomfort, cold, and tingling sensations, then this application is considered safe.

CONTRAINDICATIONS AND WHY

Contraindication	Why?
Acute pulmonary edema	Intermittent compression causes the movement of fluids through the circulatory system. If the system is already compromised, this application is not considered safe.
Acute localized infection	A localized infection can be spread through the circulatory system if intermittent compression is applied to the treatment area.
Congestive heart failure	Intermittent compression causes the movement of fluids through the circulatory system. If the system is already compromised, this application is not considered safe.
Acute deep vein thrombosis without medical management and follow-up	Compression is intended to cause the movement of fluids. A thrombus may become dislodged and move to the heart, lungs, or brain, causing additional complications.

LAB ACTIVITIES

Edema Assessment Using a Tape Measure

1. Select two classmates/patients of different body sizes. You will take circumferential measurements of their right and left upper extremities. Position the patients so that they are supine, with the extremity to measure first elevated and supported. For you to measure the extremity, you will need to support both the distal and proximal aspects.

2. Clean the tape measure with alcohol. Using a pen, place a mark on the medial aspect of the forearm at the level of the styloid process of the ulna. Place another mark at the bicipital crease of the elbow.

3. Using the tape measure, place a mark on the skin every 1½ inches moving proximally to the axilla from the elbow and distally every ½ inch to the wrist (Fig. 7-1). A small mark is preferred as some inks may cause allergic reactions or injure fragile skin.

4. Record your and your partner's measurements in the table below. Start with the distal measurements and work proximally.

Your measurements	R	L	R	L	R	L	R	L	R	L
Partner's measurements	R	L	R	L	R	L	R	L	R	L

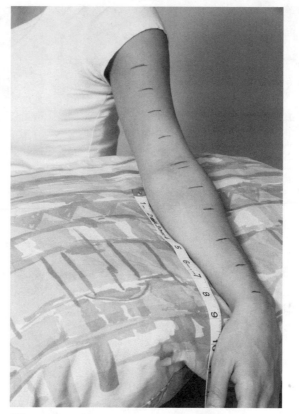

Figure 7-1 Upper extremity with markings made every 1½ inches starting from the styloid process of the radius and moving proximally.

5. Have another one of your classmates perform the same measurements and compare their measurements to those that you recorded.

Your measurements	R	L	R	L	R	L	R	L	R	L
Partner's measurements	R	L	R	L	R	L	R	L	R	L

6. Switch places with the patients and repeat the process of measurement. Compare your findings.

Edema Assessment With a Volumeter

1. Select two classmates/patients who will have the volume of their feet and ankles assessed with a volumeter.

2. Fill the volumeter with water to the "start line." The water should be warm (above 99°F [37°C]). Record the temperature of the water (Fig. 7-2).

Water Temperature: _____

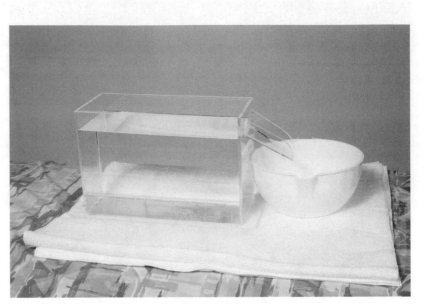

Figure 7-2 Water-filled volumeter with a water catch basin placed underneath the spout.

3. Inspect the foot to be immersed. Make sure that it is clean and there are no open lesions.

4. Position the catch basin so that it is below the spout of the volumeter (Fig. 7-3).

5. Have the patient stand so that his or her foot is flat on the bottom of the volumeter. Water will flow out the spout into the basin (Figs. 7-4 through 7-6).

6. Have the patient remove his or her foot and resume sitting on a treatment table.

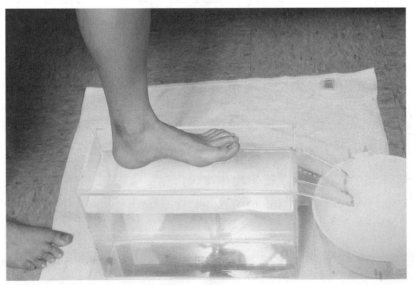

Figure 7-3 The standing patient is about to lower her foot and ankle into the water-filled volumeter.

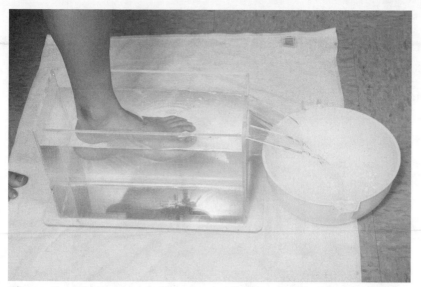

Figure 7-4 The patient is lowering her foot and ankle into the water-filled volumeter. The catch basin is collecting the displaced water.

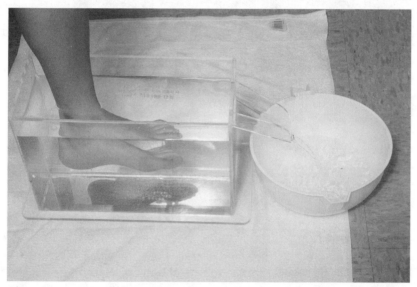

Figure 7-5 The patient is lowering her foot and ankle into the water-filled volumeter. The catch basin continues to collect the displaced water.

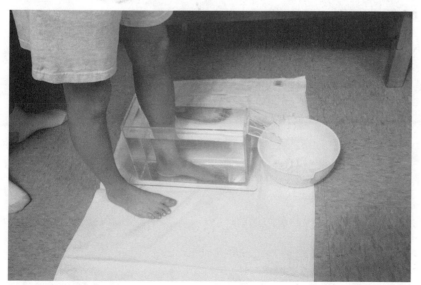

Figure 7-6 The plantar surface of the patient's foot is in contact with the bottom of the volumeter.

7. Measure and record the volume of displaced water using a graduated cylinder (Figs. 7-7 and 7-8).

    Volume: _____

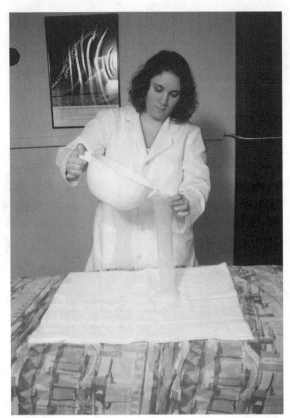

Figure 7-7 The clinician takes the water catch basin to measure the volume of water displaced.

8. Empty the water, clean the volumeter, and refill it. Repeat these steps, but this time use cold water, approximately 40°F.

9. Record your measurements and observations.

    Water Temperature: _____

    Volume: _____

    Observations: _____

    _____

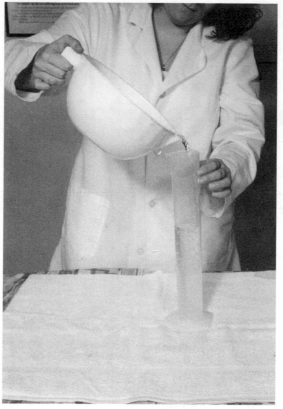

Figure 7-8 The displaced water is measured in a graduated cylinder to determine the volume.

Orientation to Intermittent Compression Devices

1. Read the instruction manual for the device. Locate the controls on the device that will adjust the inflation pressure, the deflation pressure, on time, off time, and treatment time. Select a classmate/patient to receive intermittent compression to the lower extremity.

2. Position and drape the patient so that they will be comfortable during the procedure. Inspect the extremity for open lesions, hematomas, etc.

3. Measure the extremity from the knee to about 9 inches proximal to the knee using the same technique as for the upper extremity (Figs. 7-9 and 7-10).

4. Record your and your partner's measurements in the table below. Start with the distal measurements and work proximally.

Your Measurements										
	R	L	R	L	R	L	R	L	R	L
Pretreatment										
	R	L	R	L	R	L	R	L	R	L
Posttreatment										
	R	L	R	L	R	L	R	L	R	L
Difference										

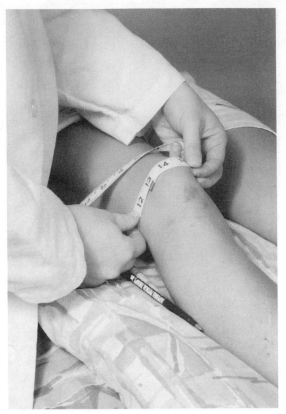

Figure 7-9 Circumferential measurement of the superior aspect of the knee is made using a tape measure.

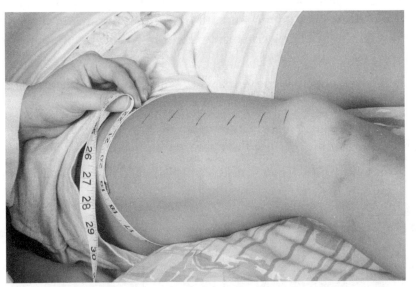

Figure 7-10 Sequential markings are placed on the thigh every 1½ inches starting at the superior border of the patella and moving proximally.

Your Partner's Measurements										
	R	L	R	L	R	L	R	L	R	L
Pretreatment										
	R	L	R	L	R	L	R	L	R	L
Posttreatment										
	R	L	R	L	R	L	R	L	R	L
Difference										

5. Monitor and check the pedal and popliteal pulses. Record your observations.

_____

_____

6. Take and record the resting heart rate and blood pressure.

Resting Heart Rate: _____

_____

Resting Blood Pressure: _____

_____

7. Apply a stockinette to the extremity. Make sure that there are no folds or creases.

8. Apply the lower extremity appliance. Re-check the patient's position and ensure that the leg is elevated and supported (Figs. 7-11 and 7-12).

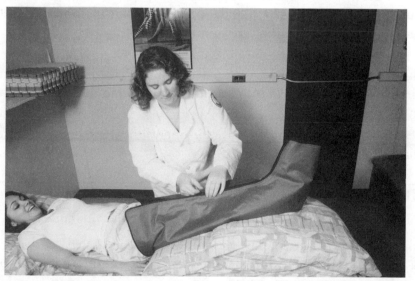

Figure 7-11 The clinician ensures that there are no wrinkles within the appliance and that the patient is properly positioned for application of intermittent compression to the lower extremity.

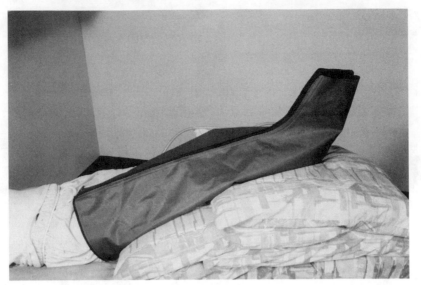

Figure 7-12 The patient's lower extremity is positioned for intermittent compression with pillows to assist in elevating the distal extent of the limb.

9. Check the inflation and deflation pressures on the device. Set the inflation pressure to 50 mm Hg and the deflation pressure to 20 mm Hg.

> **Special Considerations When Administering Intermittent Compression**
>
> • Inflation pressure must be kept below the patient's diastolic pressure so that vessels are not occluded during the compression phase.
> • Patients must be encouraged to move fingers and toes during the off times to encourage circulation in the distal extremities.

10. Set the on time to 20 seconds and off time to 6 seconds. (If you cannot individually set these parameters or the device has preset parameters, select the preset that is closest to this ratio, and record your settings.)

11. Start the device. Stay until the inflation is complete and the device has gone through two complete cycles. Let the device run for 15 minutes. Check the patient to make sure that they are comfortable.

12. Once the time is up, deflate the appliance, remove the appliance, remove the stockinette, and quickly re-measure the extremity. Record your posttreatment findings and observations in the chart in question 3 and calculate the differences, if any.

13. Repeat so that other classmates have the opportunity to feel the compression appliance as it inflates and deflates.

▉ PATIENT SCENARIOS

Read through the patient scenarios and determine the following for each:

• Whether or not intermittent compression would be indicated
• If you decided that it was not indicated due to a lack of information, what additional information you would need to know
• If indicated, what a realistic expectation of the treatment would be
• If indicated, how treatment would be applied

- patient position
- patient instruction
- additional considerations
- How you will assess whether or not your parameter selections were appropriate
- When intermittent compression would be contraindicated
- When edema assessment techniques should be employed
- Which edema assessment technique would be the most appropriate

A. Todd has been referred to therapy for an injury to his left ankle as a result of his falling from a ladder. He works as a roofer. His ankle is now edematous, particularly anterior to the lateral malleolus. Todd fell 3 weeks ago, but didn't seek medical attention until now because he didn't want to miss work. No fractures were noted by the physician. Todd has a long history of ankle sprains and strains, approximately one per year for the past 10 years. Other than being diabetic, he has no other significant medical history. His chief complaint is that he is unable to wear his work boots due to the swelling. He has no complaints of pain.

B. Karen is a legal secretary who was referred to therapy for lymphedema secondary to a radical mastectomy on the left. Karen was diagnosed with breast cancer approximately 6 months ago. Since the surgery, she has had bouts of depression and has been unable to work. She is now undergoing chemotherapy, and her physician has assured her that there were no signs of active cancer in the surrounding tissues. Her left arm is so edematous that she has difficulty lifting it, which makes work impossible.

C. Inga is a hairdresser who has been having a great deal of difficulty with fluid retention in both legs. She is on her feet all day and rarely has a chance to sit down. She is 5 months pregnant with her first child. Inga has been referred to therapy for edema reduction. She has no significant medical history.

D. Keith is a college student who is returning to school after retiring from another career. He has three grown children who live with him and his wife. One of his daughters is pregnant, and she has been having a difficult time with the pregnancy. Keith is obese and has a classic "Type A" personality. Thus far, his GPA is a 4.0. Keith saw a physician because of the sudden accumulation of fluids in all his extremities.

◼ DOCUMENTATION

Because there are different techniques for the assessment of edema, it is important to document the technique used. In addition, edema is a cyclic event, which means that it is important to re-examine the patient at the same time of the day for every session. It is helpful to record comparisons with the unaffected extremity to note differences.

If the patient is taking a diuretic, this may skew measurements and should be noted in the documentation. Sudden weight gains or losses (10 lb or more) should be noted because they may relate to fluid retention. Changes in treatment regimen should also be noted because this may affect fluid retention.

Intermittent compression may be an effective treatment tool for the patient. For there to be sustained benefit, it may be necessary for the patient to have greater access to the device, as in a rental. If the patient will be using a device, care must be taken to ensure that the patient is fully aware of the operation of the device and familiar with potential problems that may arise. Additionally, the parameters for the device must be clearly spelled out for the patient to refer to at home.

- Whether the patient uses a device outside of the department setting or receives treatment in the clinic, it is important to document the settings of the device.
- Periodic measurements should be taken to document progress or lack thereof.
- The method of measurement must be consistent so comparisons can be made. For example, if volumetric measurements were used initially, then they should be used for periodic re-evaluation of the edema. *SAME PLACE OF MEASURE*
- Patient response to the application of the device should also be recorded. Some patients may experience an increased urgency to urinate after intermittent compression. This should be documented. If fluid intake and output are monitored by nursing staff, then plans should include the measurement of urine produced following intermittent compression.

The documentation must include the following information:

- Resting heart rate *— Pulse   before you stand up from bed*
- Resting blood pressure
- Inflation pressure
- Deflation pressure
- On and off times
- Total treatment time
- Extremity treated

◼ LAB QUESTIONS

1. What is the rationale for marking off the bicipital crease as a starting point for measurement of the upper extremity?
2. What potential reasons are there for using a vinyl tape measure?
3. Of what potential significance is hand dominance in the assessment of edema? Were there differences between your dominant and nondominant hand?
4. What is the potential reason for differences in the measurements that you took and that another classmate recorded?
5. If you noted differences, how will you address this in the future and what does it mean to your practice?
6. Why does the time of day make a difference in edema measurements?
7. What information does the tape measure provide that the volumeter does not?
8. What information does the volumeter provide that the tape measure does not?
9. Was there any difference in the volumeter readings for the warm water versus the cold water? Why or why not?
10. What sensations did the patient report while the intermittent compression device was operating?
11. Were there any differences between pretreatment and posttreatment measurements? What explains this?
12. What is the rationale for a deflation pressure on this type of device?
13. Why were relatively low pressures used? Why not use a pressure that more closely resembles the blood pressure of the patient?
14. What explains the connection between urination and edema?

Foundations of Electrical Stimulation

PURPOSE

This lab activity is designed to familiarize student/learners with the common terminology associated with electrical stimulation devices. There are a wide variety of adjustable parameters and often several names for the same parameter. Student/learners will be guided through a familiarization process with the devices, and then they will apply electrodes to each other and adjust individual parameters.

This lab activity is not intended to demonstrate specific electrode placement sites for the accomplishment of therapeutic goals. It is an informal practice session and is intended to foster a minimum comfort level with electrical stimulation devices.

OBJECTIVES

Following the completion of this lab activity the student/learner will be able to:

- Differentiate between the available parameters of electrical stimulation devices and describe the differences among them to a peer
- Describe the relationships between technical terminology and sensory responses to electrical stimulation and accurately match each term with the sensation that it produces
- Describe the principles behind the application of electrodes for electrical stimulation to elicit a comfortable level of stimulation and discuss what can be done to improve patient comfort
- Demonstrate the adjustment of various parameters on electrical stimulation devices to intentionally elicit sensory, motor, and fast pain responses and accurately document the parameters so that the response can be duplicated by a peer

EQUIPMENT THAT YOU WILL NEED (FIGS. 8-1 THROUGH 8-3)

electrical stimulation devices (portable and clinical models with adjustable parameters)
1 pair large electrodes
1 pair small electrodes

conductive interface samples (eg, self-adhering, sponge, gel) for each pair of electrodes
straps to secure electrodes

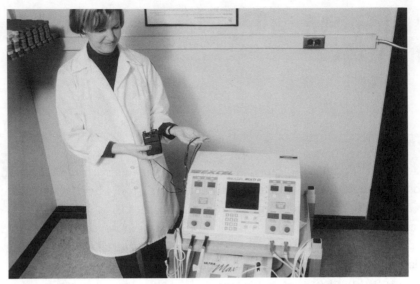

Figure 8-1 Clinician holding a portable electrical stimulator in her hand while standing next to a clinical stimulator.

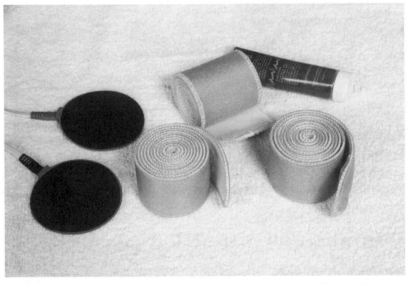

Figure 8-2 Electrodes, straps, and electrically conductive gel that can be used on the electrodes to promote conductivity.

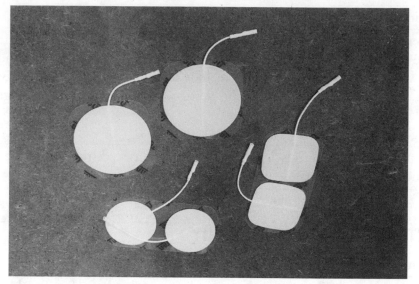

Figure 8-3 Three different sizes of self-adhering reusable electrodes.

PRECAUTIONS AND WHY

Precaution	Why?
Unstable fracture	If electrical stimulation is used for a motor response, this is a contraindication. However, if no motor response is elicited, electrical stimulation can be considered safe.
Decreased sensation	If the desired response is dependent on sensation, then electrical stimulation may be useless. However, if the desired response relies on a motor response, then the application may be considered safe.
	If the application involves the transmission of ions through the skin, the patient must be able to report sensation to avoid an adverse response.
Impaired cognitive ability	If the desired response is dependent on sensation, then electrical stimulation may be useless. However, if the desiredresponse relies on a motor response, then the application may be considered safe.
	If the application involves the transmission of ions through the skin, the patient must be able to report sensation to avoid an adverse response.
Pregnancy	If the application is after the first trimester, there is little risk to the fetus or the patient. Electrical stimulation has been safely used for analgesia during labor and delivery, but it may interfere with fetal monitors.
Heart problems (suspected or diagnosed)	Vital signs should be closely monitored before, during, and after treatment for potential changes.

Precaution	Why?
Documented evidence of epilepsy, cerebral vascular accident, or reversible ischemic neurologic deficit	Patients should be monitored carefully when electrical stimulation is used in the cervical region. Possible adverse responses may include temporary change in cognitive status, headache, vertigo, and other neurological signs.
Recent surgical procedure	A muscle contraction may cause a disruption in the healing process.

◼ CONTRAINDICATIONS AND WHY

Contraindication	Why?
Pregnancy (first trimester)	There is no data to indicate the level of safety for the fetus with the application of electrical stimulation during the first trimester of pregnancy.
Over the carotid sinus	If the circulation to the brain was altered, there could be adverse effects.
Pacemaker	Electrical stimulation devices may interfere with the electrical demands of the pacemaker.
Cancerous lesions	Most application techniques have the potential to produce an increase in circulation to the area. The possibility exists that electrical stimulation over or in proximity to cancerous lesions may enhance the development of metastasis.

◼ LAB ACTIVITIES

Orientation to Electrical Stimulation Equipment

1. Select an electrical stimulator and identify and record the following information.

   Name of Stimulator: _Excell Mult, III_

   Manufacturer: _lat . S. Medical L.L.C._

   No. of Lead Wires: _4_

   No. of Available Channels: _4_

2. Identify the controls on your stimulator. Other words may be used to identify these controls; circle those that you find on the unit that you examine. (Not all stimulators will have all of these controls.)

- Frequency Rate, PPS, Hertz, CPS, Carrier, Burst

  _____

- Intensity (mAmp, V)

  _____

  _____

- On/Off Times

  Contract / Rest

  _____

  _____

- Pulse Duration

  _____

  _____

- Reciprocal (simultaneous, alternating)

  _____

  _____

3. Inspect the electrodes that you will use and record your observations. (Are they cracked, shiny, uniformly covered? How many electrodes attach to the lead wire?)

   Self adhesive electrode, brand new very stickly. 2 electrodes per lead wire

4. There are several common forms of lead wires and electrodes used in the clinic. For electrical stimulation to take place, there need to be at least two electrodes in contact with a conductive interface and the patient. These two electrodes must be from one channel of the stimulator. Circle which of the following types of lead/pin set-ups you have on the stimulator that you selected (Figs. 8-4 and 8-5).
   - 1, 2, or more stereo jacks
   - 1, 2, or more single-lead jacks
   - Bifurcated lead (split lead with 2 pins)
   - Pin leads (small diameter, nonadjustable)
   - Banana pins (larger diameter, adjustable)
   - Other (describe)

     _____

     _____

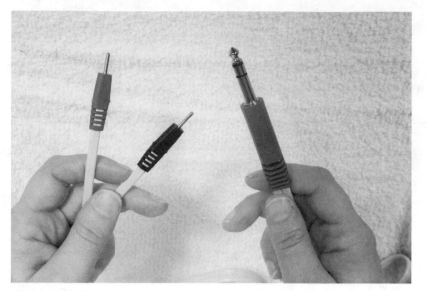

Figure 8-4 The "proximal" end of a lead wire with a stereo jack and the "distal" end with pin leads.

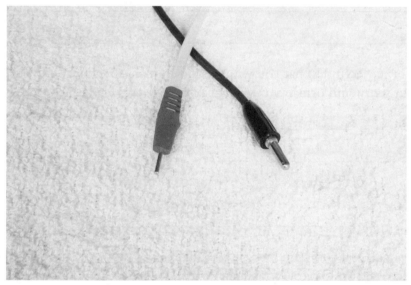

Figure 8-5 Compare the size of a pin lead on the left with a banana pin on the right.

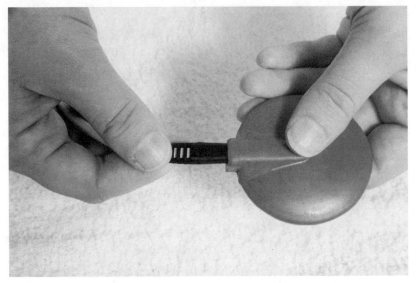

Figure 8-6 Lead wire and pin that has been inserted into an electrode.

5. Plug the leads into your electrodes so that no metal shows from the pins (Figs. 8-6 and 8-7).

Orientation to the Sensations and Responses of Electrical Stimulation Parameters

1. Select a classmate/patient to receive electrical stimulation to his or her forearm. The area should be assessed for sensation and any abnormalities such as scars or excessively dry skin or hair which may alter the conductivity of the skin.

   • Clinical models start with these three steps:
     • check the power cable for any fraying or loose wires (Fig. 8-8)
     • plug the stimulator into the wall outlet
     • turn on the power to the stimulator

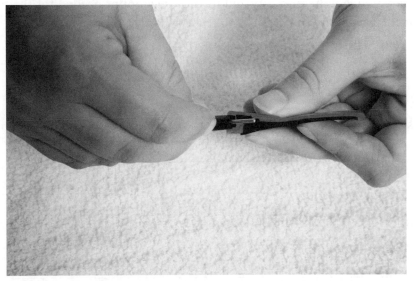

Figure 8-7 The pin from the lead wire must be fully engaged in the electrode to reach the conductive aspect of the electrode.

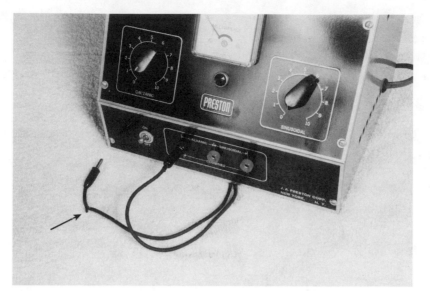

Figure 8-8 A frayed lead wire. A lead wire in this condition is considered unsafe for use.

- Portable models start with these four steps:
  - turn all outputs to zero
  - plug the leads that you will be using into the stimulator
  - prepare the electrodes for attachment to the patient (eg, wet sponges, spread gel, peel off plastic)
  - attach the electrodes to the patient (one over the wrist extensor muscle belly, one on the distal extent of the muscle belly)

2. Set the following parameters:
   - 10 minutes
   - 100 Hz (or highest available setting for that unit)
   - 200 μsec pulse duration
   - continuous on time

3. Gradually increase the intensity and record the amount needed for the patient to first start feeling something.

   10   milli amperes

- Ask the patient to describe the sensation, and record his or her response.

   Tingling initially, then prickling

- Increase the intensity until the sensation is strong but tolerable and record it. How high was it in comparison to the initial setting?

   28 milli amperes

- After 5 minutes, ask the patient to describe how the sensation has changed and record his or her response.

  feels more of a vibration

4. Decrease the intensity to zero, disconnect the electrodes from the patient, and turn off the power to the stimulator.

5. Repeat this exercise until everyone in your group has had a chance to be both the clinician and the patient.

1. Select another stimulator and familiarize yourself with the controls, leads, and electrodes.

2. Set the following parameters:
   - 15 minutes
   - 1 Hz _(20 Hz)_
   - 200 μsec pulse duration
   - continuous on time

3. Attach the electrodes to the same sites as described previously.

4. Gradually increase the intensity and record the amount needed for the patient to first start feeling something.

   11 milliamperes

   - Ask the patient to describe the sensation and record his or her response.

     Slight prickling

   - Increase the intensity until the sensation is strong but tolerable and record it. How high was it in comparison to the initial setting?

     31 milliamperes

   - After 5 minutes, ask the patient to describe how the sensation has changed and record his or her response.

     Vibrating & pulsing at the same time

5. Add a new parameter and see what changes.
   - Gradually increase the frequency. Ask the patient how the sensation changes and record his or her response.

   9 milliamperes, slight tingling

   - Increase the frequency to 50 Hz and record your observations.

   At the frequency of 50Hz, the intensity was less - 30 milliamperes

6. Decrease the intensity to zero, disconnect the electrodes from the patient, and turn off the power to the stimulator.

Mapping Your Personal Strength Duration Curve

1. Set the following parameters:
   - Pulse duration: 100 μsec *(120)*
   - Frequency: 50 pps
   - Intensity: 0
   - Continuous on time

2. Increase the intensity. At what level do you first feel something?

   More of a vibration at 10 milliamperes

3. Describe that sensation. Is it tingling, a contraction, *28* a sharp pain, or something else?

   Feels the tingling at 12 milli amperes at prox electrod and a little biting

4. Set the following parameters:
   - Pulse duration: 200 μsec *(180)*
   - Frequency: 50 pps
   - Intensity: 0
   - Continuous on time

5. Increase the intensity. At what level do you first feel something?

   9 milliamperes

26

6. Describe that sensation. Is it tingling, a contraction, a sharp pain, or something else?

More of a tingling at 14 milliamperes and vibrating

7. Set the following parameters:
   - Pulse duration: 0 μsec *(40)*
   - Frequency: 50 pps
   - Intensity: as high as possible

8. Increase the pulse duration. At what level do you first feel something?

17 feel something
20 mAmp

9. Describe that sensation. Is it tingling, a contraction, a sharp pain, or something else?

43

22 milliamperes
Tingles

10. Fill in the following chart with the data that you have collected. (Intensity is on the vertical axis, and pulse duration is on the horizontal axis.)
    - Use dots for tingling sensation
    - Use triangles for contraction
    - Use squares for sharp pain

Personal Strength Duration Curve

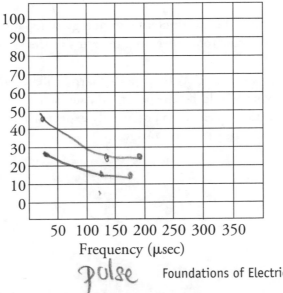

Frequency (μsec)

pulse

■ LAB QUESTIONS

1. What terms were used to describe frequency?
2. Which frequency produced a "buzzing" sensation?
3. Which frequency produced a "thumping" sensation?
4. What were the terms used to describe pulse duration?
5. What happened when the sensory level of intensity was increased above initial sensation?
6. Why was there a specific sequence for powering up and powering down the stimulators?
7. What would happen if an electrode fell off during treatment? What would the patient feel?
8. If you were treating a patient with electrical stimulation and you were utilizing a portable unit that had adjustable parameters, what would you do if the intensity was turned up as high as possible and the patient still did not feel the stimulus?
9. From your "Personal Strength Duration Curve," answer the following questions based on the information you collected.

   • Which of the sensations required the least amount of intensity to elicit?
   • Which of the sensations required the shortest pulse duration to elicit?
   • What would it mean if a patient started to have a twitching type contraction?
   • What would the minimum pulse duration be, and how high would the intensity be, and what would the frequency be?

10. When turning off an electrical stimulator, what controls should be returned to zero and why?
11. What controls may be left alone, when turning off an electrical stimulator?
12. If you were adjusting the intensity and the patient reported that they felt the current very strongly, just after you started to increase it, what would be the possible explanations for this?
13. You are increasing the intensity on a unit, and after increasing it to the maximum level, the patient still reports that they feel little or no sensation. What are the possible causes and remedies?
14. You are setting up an electrical stimulation unit and while adjusting the unit, the patient reports that they are feeling a throbbing sensation under the electrodes. What would be the possible causes for this, and what would be the remedies?
15. If you had to explain the parameter terminology to a patient, what would you say that each of the controls represents in terms of the sensations that they will feel?
16. If a patient reports to you that they feel a sharp knifelike sensation underneath the electrodes, what would be the potential causes, and remedies for this?
17. What would you tell a patient to potentially expect when you are adjusting the intensity of the stimulus to a motor level?

Electrodes: Materials and Care

9

PURPOSE

This lab activity is designed to orient student/learners to the principles of safe and efficacious use of surface electrodes for the delivery of electrical stimulation to a patient. There are different types of electrodes, electrode interfaces, and modes of electrode attachment, all of which influence the outcome of the intervention with electrical stimulation.

OBJECTIVES

Following the completion of this lab activity, the student/learner will be able to:

- Describe several different types of electrodes that can be used for the delivery of electrical stimulation to a patient and demonstrate the application of each for therapeutic purposes
- Describe the relationship between current density and the electrode interface and demonstrate how it relates to the clinical application of electrical stimulation
- Demonstrate problem-solving skills with electrodes and electrical stimulation to improve patient comfort and accomplish more predictable patient responses

EQUIPMENT THAT YOU WILL NEED

electrical stimulation unit
lead wires with 2 pin leads
electrodes
    small and large
    self-adhering
    carbon rubber

sponges to fit carbon electrodes
electrically conductive gel or lotion
water
straps to secure electrodes

PRECAUTIONS AND WHY

Precaution	Why?
Unstable fracture	If electrical stimulation is used for a motor response, this is a contraindication. However, if no motor response is elicited, electrical stimulation can be considered safe.
Decreased sensation	If the desired response is dependent on sensation, then electrical stimulation may be useless. However, if the desired response relies on a motor response, then the application may be considered safe. If the application involves the transmission of ions through the skin, the patient must be able to report sensation to avoid an adverse response.

Precaution	Why?
Impaired cognitive ability	If the desired response is dependent on sensation, then electrical stimulation may be useless. However, if the desird response relies on a motor response, then the application may be considered safe. If the application involves the transmission of ions through the skin, the patient must be able to report sensation to avoid an adverse response.
Pregnancy	If the application is after the first trimester, there is little risk to the fetus or the patient. Electrical stimulation has been safely used for analgesia during labor and delivery, but it may interfere with fetal monitors.
Heart problems (suspected or diagnosed)	Vital signs should be closely monitored before, during, and aftertreatment for potential changes.
Documented evidence of epilepsy, cerebral vascular accident, or reversible ischemic neurologic deficit	Patients should be monitored carefully when electrical stimulation is used in the cervical region. Possible adverse responses may include temporary change in cognitive status, headache, vertigo, and other neurological signs.
Recent surgical procedure	A muscle contraction may cause a disruption in the healing process.

▉ CONTRAINDICATIONS AND WHY

Contraindication	Why?
Pregnancy (first trimester)	There is no data to indicate the level of safety for the fetus with the application of electrical stimulation during the first trimester of pregnancy.
Over the carotid sinus	If the circulation to the brain was altered, there could be adverse effects.
Pacemaker	Electrical stimulation devices may interfere with the electrical demands of the pacemaker.
Cancerous lesions	Most application techniques have the potential to produce an increase in circulation to the area. The possibility exists that electrical stimulation over or in proximity to cancerous lesions may enhance the development of metastasis.

Orientation to Electrode Interfaces

Self-Adhering Electrodes

1. Select a classmate/patient to receive electrical stimulation to his or her forearm. The area should be assessed for sensation and any abnormalities such as scars or excessively dry skin or hair which may alter the conductivity of the skin.

2. Select two self-adhering electrodes of equal size. Plug the lead wires into the electrodes and into the stimulator. Set the stimulator with the following parameters:
    *   Frequency: 120 Hz
    *   Pulse Duration: Short (lowest setting on the unit) *(Phase time)*

3. Apply one electrode to the patient's forearm over the muscle belly of the wrist extensors. Apply the other electrode over the distal extent of the muscle belly, just proximal to the tendon (Fig. 9-1).

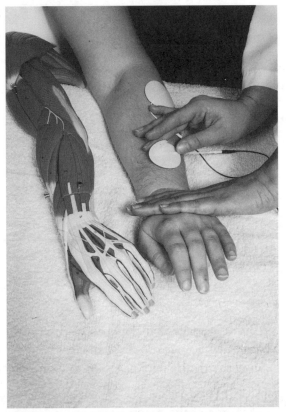

Figure 9-1 Electrode placement sites for wrist extensors using equally sized electrodes.

4. Gradually increase the intensity, and record the amount needed for the patient to begin feeling something.

    At 14 milliampere, pt felt something

    *   Ask the patient to describe the sensation, and record his or her response.

    At 13 milliampers, pt felt a light tingling

5. Turn the stimulator off, and mark where the electrodes were placed on the patient.

6. Repeat the steps that you just completed but this time, moisten the electrodes first by dipping your fingers in a cup of water and rubbing them over the surface of the electrodes.

7. Attach the electrodes to the same sites as described previously.

8. Gradually increase the intensity, and record the amount needed for the patient to begin feeling something.

   Feel the sensation at 13 milli amperes

   - Ask the patient to describe the sensation, and record his or her response.

     Slightly stronger Tingling or prickling

9. Turn the stimulator off, and remove the electrodes from the patient. Replace the protective plastic over the surface of the electrodes.

10. Was there a difference in the intensity necessary to elicit a response once the electrodes were wet? Why or why not?

    Yes, there is a slight difference in the intensity

Non–Self-Adhering Carbon Electrodes

Carbon electrodes have the advantage that they can be used many times and tend to be cost effective. However, they do need to have an electrically conductive interface and must make good contact with the patient's skin to work effectively.

1. Select two carbon electrodes that are the same size as the self-adhering electrodes that you used for the previous activity and obtain the corresponding sponges to fit them. Sponge should extend beyond the border of the carbon electrode (Fig. 9-2).

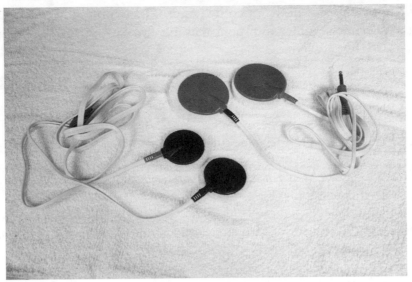

Figure 9-2 The sponge extends beyond the border of the carbon electrode.

2. Moisten the electrodes by fully submersing them in water and wringing them out so that some moisture remains but not enough to leave a trail of water dripping from under the sponge.

3. Secure the electrodes using the straps so that there is enough pressure to maintain even contact under the electrode but not so much pressure that circulation to the part is compromised (Fig. 9-3).

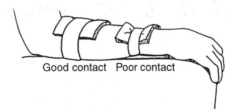

Good contact   Poor contact

Figure 9-3 Straps may be used to secure carbon electrodes and sponges. It is important to make sure that there is enough pressure to maintain even contact under the electrode but not so much pressure that circulation is compromised.

4. Gradually increase the intensity and record the amount needed for the patient to begin feeling something.

   At 14 milliamperes, she felt slight sensation

   • Ask the patient to describe the sensation, and record his or her response.

   Very slight sensation

5. Was there a difference in the intensity required to accomplish the same sensation with the carbon electrodes and sponges as there was with the self-adhering electrodes? Why or why not?

Yes, with the carbon electrode there is a very slig slight sensation, with self-adhesive is a little stronger, sensation because if it has more contact w/ the skin than carbon electrodes & sponges

6. Select the same size carbon electrodes you used for the previous activity. Cover the surface of the electrodes with electrically conductive gel before placing them on the surface of the skin.

7. Secure the electrodes with tape, but be sure that the patient is not allergic to the tape that you are using. It is also a good idea to be cautious with tape because some products stick so well to the integument that they may harm the skin when removed. Additionally, the adhesive may be difficult to remove from the surface of the carbon electrode and sometimes migrates on to the conductive surface of the electrode, which then decreases the current density of the conductive interface.

8. Gradually increase the intensity and record the amount needed for the patient to begin feeling something.

Felt the prickling sensation at 12 which is more than the carbon electrode & sponge.

   • Ask the patient to describe the sensation, and record his or her response.

   _____

   _____

9. Was there a difference in the intensity required to accomplish the same sensation with the carbon electrodes and electrically conductive gel as there was with the self-adhering electrodes? With the carbon electrodes and sponges? Why or why not?

Yes, there was less intensity with the gel than carbon electrode and sponge.

   _____

Orientation to Current Density

1. You previously used two equally sized electrodes. Set up a lead wire so that one electrode is less than half the size of the other electrode on that channel. Place the smaller electrode over the center of the muscle belly and the other electrode distal on the muscle belly, as previous (Fig. 9-4).

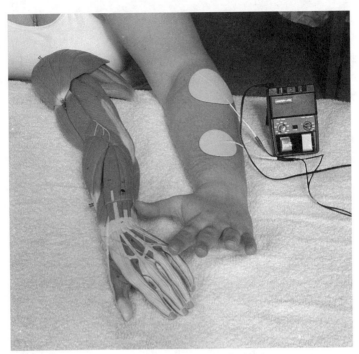

Figure 9-4 Electrode placement sites for wrist extensors using electrodes of different sizes. The proximal electrode is larger than the distal electrode.

2. Gradually increase the intensity, and record the patient's responses.

   7 milliamperes

   • Does he or she feel the stimulation underneath both electrodes?

   Yes

   • Is that stimulation equally perceived under both electrodes?

   Feels slightly stronger on the proximal electrode (motor unit)

3. Gradually increase the intensity, and record the patient's responses.

   More tingling & slight move on hand
   28 milliamperes causes fingers to stand up

- Does he or she feel the stimulation underneath both electrodes?

  Yes

- If not, which one is perceived as stronger? Why?

  Pt feel stronger tingling on the motor unit electrode

4. Reverse the electrode set-up by moving the smaller electrode to the distal extent of the muscle belly and placing the larger electrode over the center of the muscle belly (Fig. 9-5).

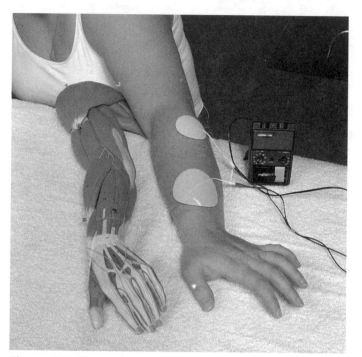

Figure 9-5 Electrode placement sites for wrist extensors using electrodes of different sizes. The proximal electrode is smaller than the distal electrode.

5. Gradually increase the intensity, and record the patient's responses.

   Pt felt tingling sensation on the ulnar side

- Does he or she feel the stimulation underneath both electrodes?

  The smaller electrode (proximal) had stronger tingling or current flow

- Is that stimulation equally perceived under both electrodes?

  No

6. Gradually increase the intensity, and record the patient's responses.

   Ulnar deviation was showed

- Does he or she feel the stimulation underneath both electrodes?

  Yes

- If not, which one is perceived as stronger? Why?

  None

◼ PATIENT SCENARIOS

Read through the patient scenarios and determine the following for each:

- Whether or not electrical stimulation could potentially be beneficial for them, and how.
- What goals could it potentially used to accomplish, and how.
- The electrode placement sites and what type of electrodes you would suggest, and why?
- The problems you could potentially expect to encounter and how you could prevent these from happening?

A. Annie is a 50-year-old secretary who has been referred to physical therapy for treatment to relieve symptoms associated with an automobile accident that she was involved in 3 weeks ago. She is having difficulty maintaining an upright posture because of severe headaches, back pain, and intermittent paresthesias in her dominant right hand. She is a frail woman who previously taught aerobics classes 5 nights a week. She is unable to teach at all now, which is adding to her stress level. There were no fractures, and she is otherwise healthy. Her chief complaints include decreased cervical ROM, muscle guarding, and pain with all active cervical motion.

B. Sam is an athletic trainer for the track team of a local high school. He has been referred to physical therapy for pain, stiffness, weakness, and edema reduction for his left ankle, which has been sprained for a total of six times in the past 3 years. His attempts at icing the joint have not been successful in reducing the edema. He has lateral instability and marked weakness in the ankle invertors and evertors on the left. Sam is motivated and has no significant medical history.

C. Fred is an avid cyclist who was recently involved in an automobile accident while riding his bike. He sustained a midshaft femoral fracture, numerous contusions and abrasions, and a cervical and lumbar strain. His lower left extremity is in a cast, and he is ambulating non–weight-bearing on the left leg with crutches. His primary complaints are of severe headaches and an inability to hold his head up while typing or trying to work at his desk. He is a college professor.

LAB QUESTIONS

1. What are the advantages to using self-adhering electrodes for electrical stimulation?
2. What are the disadvantages to using self-adhering electrodes for electrical stimulation?
3. Why would you select one type of electrode over another?
4. What is meant by the term "current density," and how does it apply to electrical stimulation?
5. How can you use your knowledge of current density to your advantage to accomplish a treatment goal with electrical stimulation?

Neuromuscular Electrical Stimulation

10

◤ PURPOSE

This lab activity builds on previously experienced electrically induced motor responses. Stimulation parameters and electrode placement sites for motor responses are different than for other treatment goals. This lab activity centers on the sensory differences as well as the importance of accurate descriptions of these sensations when instructing patients what they should and should not feel during stimulation.

◤ OBJECTIVES

Following the completion of this lab activity, the student/learner will be able to:

- Integrate the understanding of the application of specific treatment parameters with the accomplishment of specific treatment goals, and discuss which parameter sets are used to accomplish those treatment goals
- Integrate the concepts of appropriate electrode placement site selection with the accomplishment of specific treatment goals, and demonstrate the electrode placement sites necessary to accomplish those treatment goals
- Compare electrical stimulation parameters and electrode placement sites for edema reduction, muscle spasm reduction, and muscle strengthening, and demonstrate each application

◤ EQUIPMENT THAT YOU WILL NEED (FIGS. 10-1 AND 10-2)

clinical and portable electrical stimulation units with adjustable parameters
> pulse duration
> frequency
> intensity
> ramps

electrodes and lead wires appropriate for the electrical stimulation units

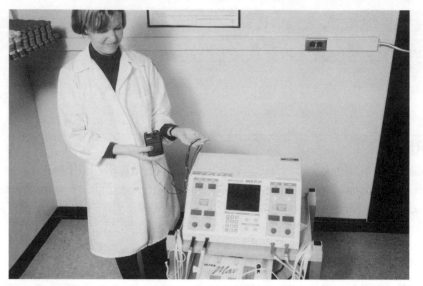

Figure 10-1 A clinician holds a portable model of an electrical stimulation unit in her hand. She is standing next to a clinical model of an electrical stimulation unit with multiple channels of stimulation that is "line operated," meaning that the unit plugs into the wall for power.

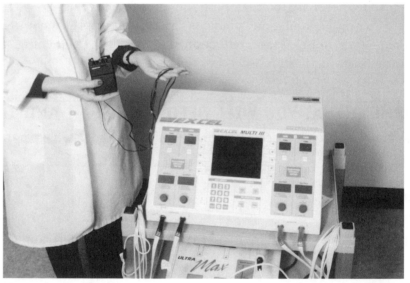

Figure 10-2 On closer inspection of clincial and portable models of electrical stimulation units, it is clear that the sizes of the lead wires for the two units are different and would not be interchangeable.

PT is an Evidence based practice!

PRECAUTIONS AND WHY

Precaution	Why?
Unstable fracture	If electrical stimulation is used for a motor response, this is a contraindication. However, if no motor response is elicited, electrical stimulation can be considered safe.
Decreased sensation	If the desired response is dependent on sensation, then electrical stimulation may be useless. However, if the desired response relies on a motor response, then the application may be considered safe. If the application involves the transmission of ions through the skin, the patient must be able to report sensation to avoid an adverse response.
Impaired cognitive ability	If the desired response is dependent on sensation, then electrical stimulation may be useless. However, if the desired response relies on a motor response, then the application may be considered safe. If the application involves the transmission of ions through the skin, the patient must be able to report sensation to avoid an adverse response.
Pregnancy	If the application is after the first trimester, there is little risk to the fetus or the patient. Electrical stimulation has been safely used for analgesia during labor and delivery, but it may interfere with fetal monitors.
Documented evidence of epilepsy, cerebral vascular accident, or reversible ischemic neurologic deficit	Patients should be monitored carefully when electrical stimulation is used in the cervical region. Possible adverse responses may include temporary change in cognitive status, headache, vertigo, and other neurological signs.

CONTRAINDICATIONS AND WHY

Contraindication	Why?
Pregnancy (first trimester)	There is no data to indicate the level of safety for the fetus with the application of electrical stimulation during the first trimester of pregnancy.
Over the carotid sinus	If the circulation to the brain was altered, there could be adverse effects.
Pacemaker	Electrical stimulation devices may interfere with the electrical demands of the pacemaker.
Cancerous lesions	Most application techniques have the potential to produce an increase in circulation to the area. The possibility exists that electrical stimulation over or in proximity to cancerous lesions may enhance the development of metastasis.

■ LAB ACTIVITIES

Eliciting Motor Responses to Electrical Stimulation

Cautions When Working With Motor Levels of Electrical Stimulation

- Do not increase the intensity during the off time. When the on time resumes, this could result in a "surprise" for the patient, which would be uncomfortable.
- Provide the patient with the emergency stop button, if applicable, or at a minimum, provide a method for him or her to contact you if needed during the unattended portion of the treatment time.
- Remember that electrode size influences the ease of eliciting a comfortable muscle contraction. Large electrodes generally have lower resistance levels, which translate into lower intensities necessary to elicit a muscle contraction.

Dorsiflexors and Plantarflexors of the Ankle

1. Select a classmate/patient for electrical stimulation to elicit a motor response in his or her calf. Position the patient as if he or she had an acutely sprained, edematous ankle (Fig. 10-3).

2. Determine where the electrodes should be placed to elicit muscle contractions in the tibialis anterior (Fig. 10-4).

3. Select a stimulator capable of producing levels of stimulation that elicit a tetanic muscle contraction. Preset the following parameters:

   - Pulse Duration: ≥200 μsec
   - Frequency: 50 Hz
   - On/Off Times: 10/10 (adjustable in seconds)
   - Reciprocal Stimulation: Yes/no

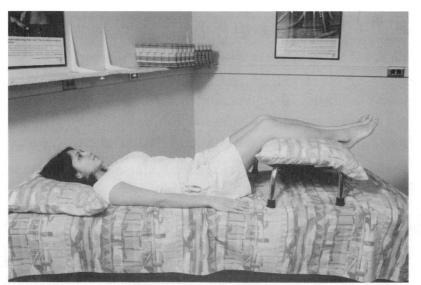

Figure 10-3 Appropriate patient positioning for an acutely sprained edematous ankle.

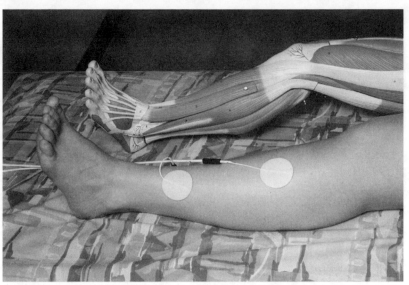

Figure 10-4 Electrode placement sites to elicit muscle contraction in the tibialis anterior.

4. Prepare and apply the electrodes that you have selected. They should be appropriately sized, relative to the sizes of the muscles that you will be stimulating.

small To medium electrode

5. How much more intensity was necessary to elicit a muscle contraction than was necessary for the patient to report that a stimulus was felt?

Sensory Stim = 20 mA

59 mA for contraction of muscle

6. What happens to the quality of the contraction as you slowly increase the frequency up to 80 pps (during the on times)?

Contraction became stronger

Toes flexed w/ more water

7. What happens to the quality of the contraction as you slowly decrease the frequency down to 10 pps (during the on times)?

Decrease contraction

8. What was the optimal frequency for the muscles that you were stimulating?

62 pps

Reduction of Muscle Guarding Using Three Different Electrical Stimulation Set-Ups

Whenever an injury occurs to soft tissue, one of the natural responses that takes place is muscle guarding, which acts to protect the area from further movement or injury. Muscle guarding impedes the circulation to the area and promotes metabolite

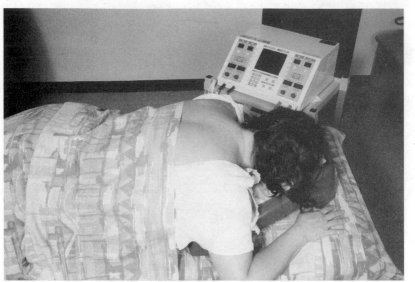

rolls on chin & forehead

Figure 10-5 Patient positioned so that she is comfortable and the upper trapezii are in a resting position.

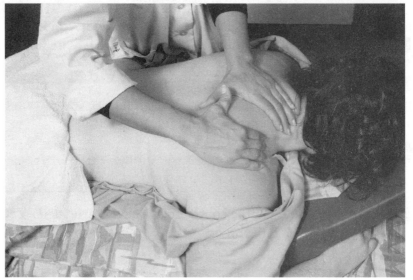

Figure 10-6 Palpation of the upper trapezii to determine the presence of increased palpable tightness or fibrous nodules.

retention. This may increase pain perception owing to the sensitization of the nociceptors by the presence of metabolic byproducts. Reduction in muscle guarding may also result in pain reduction.

1. Select a classmate/patient to receive electrical stimulation to the upper trapezius muscles bilaterally. Position the patient so that he or she is comfortable and the upper trapezii are in a resting position. If the patient has some palpable muscle tightness, assess the degree of tightness and tenderness to palpation (Figs. 10-5 and 10-6).

2. Identify the parameters that you will need to elicit a tetanic muscle contraction, and select the electrodes that you will be using. Apply the electrodes in each of the following set-up configurations: crossed (Fig. 10-7), horizontal (Fig. 10-8), and vertical (Fig. 10-9).

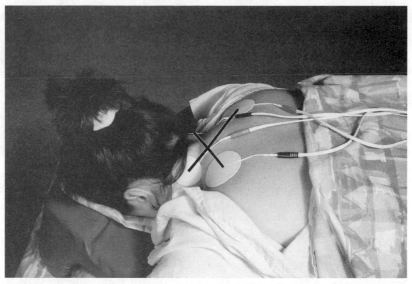

Figure 10-7 Electrode placement sites for bilateral upper traps with a crossed set-up.

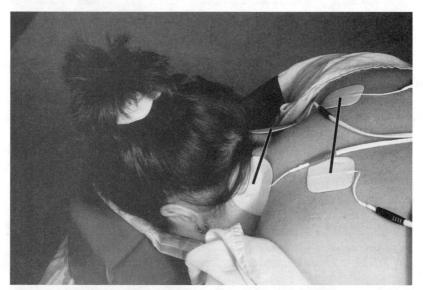

Figure 10-8 Electrode placement sites for bilateral upper traps with a horizontal set-up.

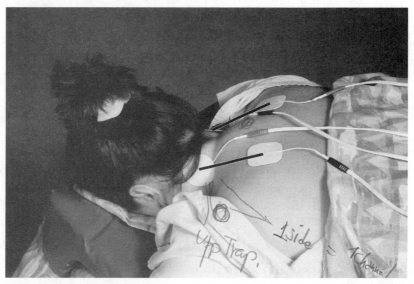

Figure 10-9 Electrode placement sites for bilateral upper traps with a vertical parallel set-up.

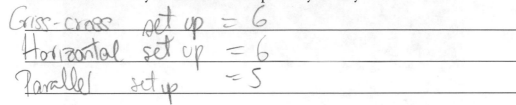

Custom Mode

continuous or
simultaneous

alternate
or

Channel 1
@ 3 on
off →

Channel #2
@ 3 off
off → on

3. First try each of the set-ups with reciprocal on/off times and 3-second on ramps. Which was the most comfortable for the patient?

Horizontal set up

4. Choose a simultaneous on time for each of the set-ups. Was there a difference in the sensation for any of the three set-ups? Why or why not?

Criss-cross set up = 6
Horizontal set up = 6
Parallel set up = 5

5. Which is more comfortable, using on ramps or not using them? Why?

Ramping more comfortable

6. If your goal is to decrease muscle guarding, specifically in the upper trapezius muscles bilaterally, which set-up would be most logical?

Criss Cross (simultaneous)

7. If your goal is to decrease the muscle's ability to maintain a contraction, what parameters would you adjust, and what would be your rationale?

Continuous Contraction to fatigue the muscle
                                          continuous
For pt w/ spasticity use constant biphasic to fatigue the mus

8. If the patient for this exercise had palpable muscle tightness before you applied the stimulation, reassess the tightness. Was there a noticeable change to you? To the patient?

No   N/A

Eliciting Motor Responses for Muscle Strengthening

Electrical stimulation has been used successfully for the enhancement of an isometric muscle contraction. It is one of the tools used in a comprehensive treatment plan for postoperative recovery after several orthopedic procedures. The key components of this form of stimulation include the isolation of the muscle group and the stabilization of the joint on which the muscle acts.

Vastus Medialis and Rectus Femoris

1. Select a classmate/patient to receive electrical stimulation of the vastus medialis and the rectus femoris.

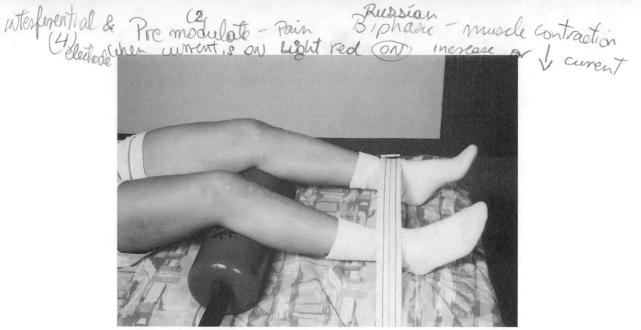

Figure 10-10 Patient positioned so that she is supported in about 20 degrees of knee flexion and no joint motion is possible.

2. Position the patient so that he or she is supported in about 20 degrees of knee flexion and no joint motion is permitted. You may use a commercial dynamometer to stabilize the joint isometrically or devise some other means to stabilize the joint (Fig. 10-10).

3. Set up the stimulator that you have selected so that you will be able to elicit strong muscle contractions. Identify electrode placement sites for both muscles, and apply the electrodes securely, one channel for each muscle (Figs. 10-11 and 10-12).

4. Slowly increase the intensity of the stimulus until a strong muscle contraction is elicited. What should the patient feel?

   A strong but comfortable contraction

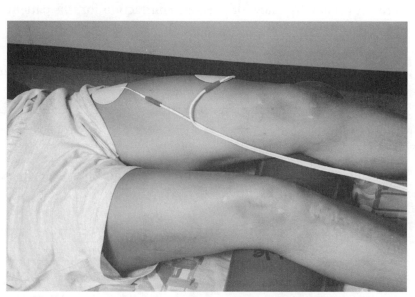

Figure 10-11 Electrode placement for the rectus femoris.

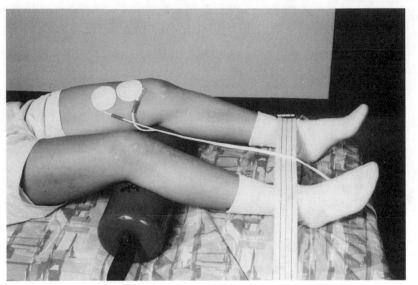

Figure 10-12 Electrode placement for the vastus medialis.

5. What would make the stimulus more comfortable for the patient?

   Gradually increase intensity / increase
   ramp time

6. Try one of your potential solutions for comfort. Does it make a difference?

   Yes, the higher the frequency, the less the
   intensity

7. How much intensity can the patient tolerate?

   _39 mA_

8. What is the optimal frequency for a tetanic contraction for this patient?

   Higher frequency more comfortable and
   low intensity are comfortable

9. What would the rationale be for a 10-second on time and 50-second off time?

   Keeps the muscle from fatigue
   slower muscle re education for the pt comfort

10. Does the quality of the muscle contraction that you are eliciting change with successive contractions? If yes, how?

    Yes Because of Acommodation of pt
    over time

11. What happens to the sensation of the stimulation if the patient contracts with the stimulation?

Make the muscle feel more comfortable when contraction occurs & intensifies electrical sensation

12. Try other options that you believe may make the stimulus more tolerable for the patient. Observe the responses. What was the "best" set-up or option for the patient?

The high frequency definitely made the stimulus more comfortable

Experiencing Functional Electrical Stimulation for Activities of Daily Living

Reduction of Shoulder Subluxation

Electrical stimulation has been used to augment muscle function in a wide variety of conditions, including urinary incontinence, shoulder subluxations, footdrop during gait, and standing stability for patients with paraplegia. One of the common elements in these applications is the development of portable "intelligent" technology that is capable of producing the necessary parameters when the patient needs them and in a way that does not interfere with a patient's ability to perform the activity itself. For example, the technology has been in existence for years to elicit a muscle contraction with electrical stimulation; however, a 6-ft power cord was usually necessary to provide the power source of stimulation. Devices are now much more portable and accessible for patients than they ever have been.

1. Select a classmate/patient to receive electrical stimulation of his or her middle deltoid and supraspinatus. You will adjust the parameters so that you can elicit a tetanic muscle contraction to help reduce a subluxation of the humeral head (Figs. 10-13 and 10-14).

2. Position the patient so that he or she will be able to see what you are doing.

3. Teach the patient the electrode placement sites that he or she will need to use and how to assess success in eliciting the desired response.

4. Familiarize yourself and the patient with the portable stimulator you will be using. Teach the patient how to inspect the treatment area and the unit, care for and apply the electrodes, and adjust the intensity controls.

5. Determine the appropriate on/off timing and whether or not on ramps are functional for this patient. Turn the unit on and have the patient set the intensity level.

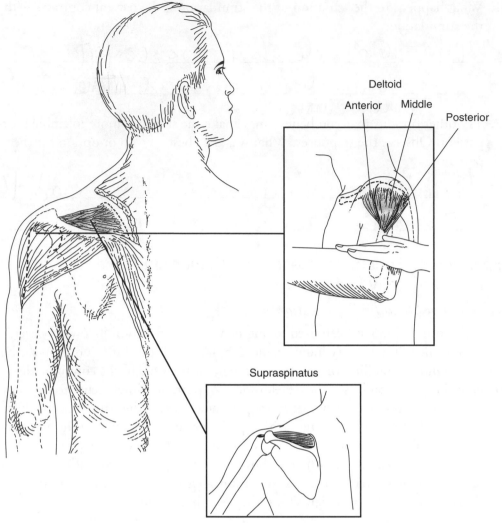

Deltoid

Anterior   Middle

Posterior

Supraspinatus

Figure 10-13 The supraspinatus and middle deltoid showing the humeral head underneath.

6. Why do you think that you were instructed to teach the patient so much during this lab activity?

To prevent skin manage and pt can operate the unit safely and put

7. How much more time did it take to teach the patient?

2 minutes no long
If the pt had questions, they were answered

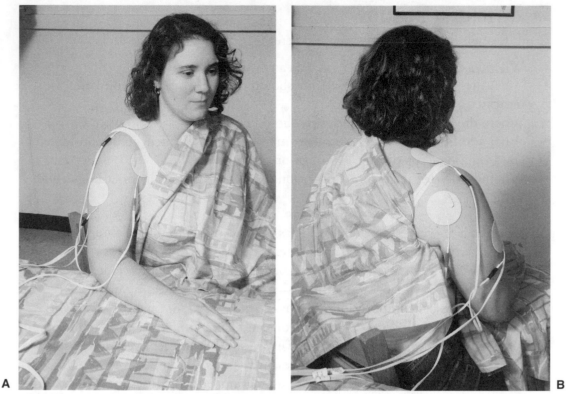

Figure 10-14 Electrode placement sites to elicit responses from both the supraspinatus and middle deltoid to approximate the humoral head. **A.** Anterior view. **B.** Posterior view.

8. What parameters did you use?

Frequency: /Rate _____ 30 _____

Pulse Duration: _____ 300 microsec (preset) _____

On/Off Times: _____ 8/24 _____
on off

Ramps: _____ 1.0 _____

Waveform: _____ Biphasic Symmetrical _____

9. Which is more important, a specific intensity reading or a specific response? Why?

_____ A specific response is more important due _____
_____ to pt comfort _____
_____
_____

■ PATIENT SCENARIOS

Read through the patient scenarios and determine the following for each:

- Whether electrical stimulation is indicated, and your rationale for your response.
- What the parameters for stimulation should be for if electrical stimulation is indicated?
- Where the electrode placement sites should be?
- What additional considerations there might be for the patient to be considered a good candidate for electrical stimulation?
- Whether the electrical stimulation should be applied clinically or at home, and why?

[handwritten: wheelchair or sitting]

A. Marge is a 55-year-old woman who has been admitted to the rehabilitation hospital subsequent to an unsuccessful attempt to reduce the effects of arteriosclerosis in her carotid arteries. She has had bilateral cerebrovascular accidents (CVAs) as a result of the procedures performed. She is otherwise healthy, with no previous medical complications. She has been referred for physical therapy to determine whether electrical stimulation can be used to reduce the subluxation of her right shoulder. She is alternatively expressively and receptively aphasic and has limited manual dexterity skills. Presently, she is not ambulatory because of balance difficulties and an inability to use her upper extremities for support with assistive devices.

[handwritten: Poor Skill on hand / Fine motor] *[handwritten: No comprehen]* *[handwritten: Difficult (contraindication)]*

B. Joe is a 48-year-old shoemaker who has been referred to the physical therapy department subsequent to a CVA. He presently has flexor spasticity in his right upper extremity and right foot-drop. His goal is ambulation without the short leg brace that he has been ambulating with for the past 3 months since the CVA.

C. Grace is a legal secretary who has been referred to the physical therapy department subsequent to injuries that she sustained in an automobile accident 3 days ago. She has a cervical strain with pronounced muscle guarding throughout the cervical spine, shown by limitations in active range of motion in all directions. She also is scheduled to have a medial meniscectomy next week. Her physician and employer are concerned about her ability to return to work after the knee surgery and want her to be as prepared as she can be preoperatively to ensure a prompt return to work. She is an aerobics instructor at night and a long-distance bicycle racer who has a race scheduled in 2 months.

[handwritten: 1st Set 2 channel / Set one channel / at a time]

D. Howard is an athletic trainer for the track team of a local high school. He has been referred to physical therapy for edema reduction for his left ankle, which has been sprained a total of six times in the last 3 years. His attempts at icing the joint have not been successful in reducing the edema. He has lateral instability and marked weakness in the ankle invertors and evertors on the left. Mike is well motivated and has no other medical complications.

[handwritten: Reciprocal / 10/10 (on/off) / .5 ramp / Russian because it elicit a muscle contraction]

[handwritten: Med Lat (1 channel each side)]

[handwritten margin notes: Final Exam Practical / Precautions! Page 218 / Look Muscle that invert & evert / Reciprocal / Lat & Med Malleolus / we want a Motor response]

■ DOCUMENTATION

Documentation of treatments rendered with electrical stimulation involves at a minimum the recording of the treatment goal for which the stimulation was applied and the result. Documentation of electrode placement sites, parameters, and stimulator used is helpful in preventing a lengthy trial-and-error period before optimal results can be achieved with a different clinician or if unusual techniques must be used to accomplish the intended results. For example, if a patient had tendon transplant surgery, it would be important to know where the electrode placement sites were located.

Once the goal is identified, the parameters to accomplish the goal and the electrode placement sites necessary should be fairly obvious to other clinicians who may be reading the documentation to duplicate the treatment rendered. However, documentation should include enough information so that any clinician could duplicate the treatment.

Select two of the classmates/patients to whom you applied modalities during the lab activity and write a progress note that includes each patient's subjective complaints, the objective information that you recorded, the physical agent that was applied, the manner of application, the response, and your assessment.

■ LAB QUESTIONS

1. What was the optimal frequency for accomplishing a tetanic contraction?
2. How did your optimal frequency compare with those of your classmates?
3. Of what significance is an optimal frequency?
4. What were some of the common factors for the applications of electrical stimulation performed during this laboratory exercise?
5. If you had two stimulators to choose from, and one had a maximum pulse duration of 100 μsec and the other stimulator had a maximum pulse duration of 200 μsec, which one would require a lower intensity to elicit a tetanic muscle contraction? Why?
6. Of what potential value are on ramps?
7. Why is it more difficult to adjust parameters other than the intensity on portable functional electrical stimulators?
8. What do you think would be the most significant barriers to the successful use of functional electrical stimulation for gait? How would you potentially overcome them?
9. What objective measures could you employ to ensure that the level of electrical stimulation consistently elicited the same level of muscle contraction response?
10. Describe the necessary parameters for electrical stimulation to maintain muscle strength.

Electrical Stimulation for Tissue Repair

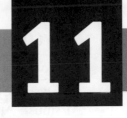

PURPOSE

This lab activity provides student/learners with the opportunity to review electrical stimulation concepts related to polarity, infection, and wound healing. Student/learners will practice problem-solving techniques with a case study that illustrates concepts related to electrical stimulation and tissue repair.

OBJECTIVES

Following the completion of this review activity, the student/learner will be able to:

- Differentiate between the effects that take place underneath the cathode and the anode when direct current electrical stimulation is applied to a patient
- Describe the potential effects of direct current on an infection in a wound
- Discuss the differences in the electrode selection process for wound care with electrical stimulation and how it differs from other applications of electrical stimulation
- Describe the stages of wound healing

PRECAUTIONS AND WHY

Precaution	Why?
Decreased sensation	If the application involves the transmission of ions through the skin, the patient must be able to report sensation to avoid an adverse response.
Impaired cognitive ability	If the application involves the transmission of ions through the skin, the patient must be able to report sensation to avoid an adverse response.
Pregnancy	If the application is after the first trimester, there is little risk to the fetus or the patient. Electrical stimulation has been safely used for analgesia during labor and delivery, but it may interfere with fetal monitors.
Documented evidence of epilepsy, cerebral vascular accident, or reversible ischemic neurologic deficit	Patients should be monitored carefully when electrical stimulation is used in the cervical region for possible adverse responses.
Heart problems (suspected or diagnosed)	Caution should be used to monitor the patient's response. Vital signs should be closely monitored before, during, and after treatment for potential changes.
Recent surgical procedure	A muscle contraction may cause a disruption in the healing process.

CONTRAINDICATIONS AND WHY

Contraindication	Why?
Over the carotid sinus	There would be potential problem if the circulation to the brain is altered.
Pacemaker	Electrical stimulation devices may interfere with the electrical demands of the pacemaker.
Metal ions from antimicrobial medications or metallic implants	Direct electrical currents may drive metal ions from antimicrobial medications into the tissues. Pulsed waveforms may result in tissue heating, which also might be inappropriate.
Pregnancy (first trimester)	There is no data to indicate the level of safety for the fetus with the application of electrical stimulation during the first trimester of pregnancy.
Cancerous lesions	Most application techniques have the potential to produce an increase in circulation to the area. The possibility exists that electrical stimulation over or in proximity to cancerous lesions may enhance the development of metastasis.

REVIEW ACTIVITIES

Polarity

1. Research the responses of tissues under an anode using three sources and develop a composite description that encompasses all of them.

   Source/Definition: _____

   _____

   Source/Definition: _____

   _____

   Source/Definition: _____

   _____

   Composite Definition: _____

   _____

   _____

2. Research the responses of tissues under a cathode using three sources and develop a composite description that encompasses all of them.

   Source/Definition: _____

   _____

Source/Definition: _____

_____

Source/Definition: _____

_____

Composite Definition: _____

_____

_____

3. What is the principal difference between using the anode or the cathode for electrical stimulation?

_____

_____

_____

_____

- When would you select the cathode?

_____

_____

- When would you select the anode?

_____

_____

4. How could this potentially be useful information for you as a clinician?

_____

_____

_____

_____

Infection

1. What is the definition of infection?

_____

_____

_____

_____

2. Based on the definition that you have written, how would the presence of and infection potentially limit healing or a return to function?

_____

_____

_____

gangrene   cancer wound   flesh eating bacteria

3. Would the presence of an infection alter your selection of the polarity of the active electrode? Why or why not?

_____

_____

_____

_____

Stages of Wound Healing

1. What are the three stages of wound/tissue healing, and approximately how long does each stage last?

_____

_____

_____

_____

2. When could electrical stimulation potentially be used to promote wound healing?

_____

_____

_____

_____

3. What special considerations would there be, if any, regarding the application of electrodes for the treatment of an open wound?

_____

_____

_____

_____

4. If you had a choice between self-adhering electrodes and saline-moistened gauze electrodes for a wound, which do you think would be more appropriate? Why?

_____

_____

_____

_____

5. Of what potential benefit would the addition of electrical stimulation for tissue repair be to the healing process?

_____

_____

_____

_____

■ CASE SCENARIO

Joan is a vivacious 67-year-old woman who has been referred to physical therapy because of the presence of a long-standing ulcer on her right calcaneus. She was treated in an inpatient setting for treatment of a hip fracture that has since healed. Before the hip fracture, she led an active lifestyle that included swimming, dancing, and sightseeing as the leader of her retirement group.

Following recovery, her lifestyle has changed specifically as a result of the development of the calcaneal ulcer that has now remained open for 2 months and measures approximately 4 cm across the widest point and at 1 cm deep. She reports that she received home care nursing without significant progress

Joan has no significant past medical history.

1. Assuming that Joan is a good candidate for electrical stimulation to help improve the possibility of accomplishing wound closure, what parameters would you select and why?

2. Where would you place your electrodes and why?

3. What instructions would you give to Joan? *I would explain her what wound are, and advance until their type of wound she has*

4. Approximately how long would you expect it to take before you see any changes— *(1 week)* in the condition of the wound, and on what do you base your response? *Monitor her every week and showed her the Q tip, rule measure, photograph, tape don't*

5. What type of changes in condition of the wound would you hope to see? *contaminate the tape / Closing wound, not as deep, edges closing together, color, odor, drainage measure*

6. What medical conditions (that Joan does not have) would have complicated this scenario? *Diabetes, congestive heart failure - edema present, arteriosclerosis, smoking, arterial insufficiency ALL blood flow deficiencies*

7. What resources could you consult to find out more information about how to proceed with application techniques for electrical stimulation for wound and tissue repair?

Textbook protocols

▰ RESOURCES

www.apta.org Section on Clinical Electrotherapy and Wound Care

www.cms.hhs.gov Centers for Medicare and Medicaid Services

www.hookedonevidence.org Hooked on Evidence, a resource database established by the American Physical Therapy Association

* Typically 7 to 10 days wound will close.

* clear & bloody is ok, no white

* swelling makes lose of sensation

* Thicker bandage to collect the drainage exudate

* Before to apply periwound Technique put pt on the 1st whirlpool w/ cloring tablets / or other pulsuvage?

Pain Management With Electrical Stimulation

PURPOSE

This lab activity is designed to familiarize the student/learner with the application and expected patient responses to transcutaneous electrical nerve stimulation (TENS) for the relief of pain. It will also familiarize the student/learner with electrode placement site selection and stimulation parameters for sensory analgesia. Student/learners will have the opportunity to experience various parameters on both portable and clinical stimulation devices.

OBJECTIVES

Following the completion of this lab activity, the student/learner will be able to:

- Describe electrode placement site selection guidelines for pain management
- Apply TENS to a patient for pain management
- Apply electrical stimulation with a clinical electrical stimulation device to accomplish sensory analgesia
- Select and adjust electrical stimulation parameters on a variety of electrical stimulation devices to accomplish pain management
- Instruct a patient in the self-application and self-adjustment of a TENS unit
- Describe the concept of interferential current (IFC) and how it differs from the application of a portable TENS unit
- Discuss the differences in electrode placement concepts with IFC and the importance of patient positioning for this modality

EQUIPMENT THAT YOU WILL NEED

TENS stimulators (clinical and portable)
    lead wires for the stimulators
    electrically conductive gel
    OR
    self-adhering electrodes
    4 equal-sized electrodes
    cloth or paper tape to secure electrodes
electrical stimulators with adjustable pulse durations
IFC stimulation unit
electrical stimulation unit with an adjustable pulse duration capable of being
    set in excess of 1 millisecond (msec)

PRECAUTIONS AND WHY

Unstable fracture	If electrical stimulation is used for a motor response, this is a contraindication. However, if no motor response is elicited, electrical stimulation can be considered safe.
Decreased sensation	If the desired response is dependent on sensation, then electrical stimulation may be useless. However, if the desired response relies on a motor response, then the application may be considered safe. If the application involves the transmission of ions through the skin, the patient must be able to report sensation to avoid an adverse response.
Impaired cognitive ability	If the desired response is dependent on sensation, then electrical stimulation may be useless. However, if the desired response relies on a motor response, then the application may be considered safe. If the application involves the transmission of ions through the skin, the patient must be able to report sensation to avoid an adverse response.
Pregnancy	If the application is after the first trimester, there is little risk to the fetus or the patient. Electrical stimulation has been safely used for analgesia during labor and delivery, but it may interfere with fetal monitors.
Documented evidence of epilepsy, cerebral vascular accident, or reversible ischemic neurologic deficit	Patients should be monitored carefully when electrical stimulation is used in the cervical region. Possible adverse responses may include temporary change in cognitive status, headache, vertigo, and other neurological signs.

CONTRAINDICATIONS AND WHY

Pregnancy (first trimester)	There is no data to indicate the level of safety for the fetus with the application of electrical stimulation during the first trimester of pregnancy.
Over the carotid sinus	If the circulation to the brain is altered, there could be adverse effects.
Pacemaker	Electrical stimulation devices may interfere with the electrical demands of the pacemaker.
Cancerous lesions	Most application techniques have the potential to produce an increase in circulation to the area. The possibility exists that electrical stimulation over or in proximity to cancerous lesions may enhance the development of metastasis.

■ LAB ACTIVITIES

Orientation to TENS Equipment

TENS Electrode Placements and Sensations

1. Familiarize yourself with the TENS device that you have selected by reviewing both the controls on the stimulator and the instruction manual for the device. You may use either a clinical or portable stimulator for this exercise. What are the available ranges of parameters?

Machine Tens

Frequency: ___1 to 80 Hz___

Pulse Duration: ___1 to 60 pps___

Intensity: ___0 to 5 Hz___

2. Are there any other controls on the device? If yes, what are they, and what do they do?

___R = Reciprocal___

___CO = Continuous___

___C = Cycle continuous___

___Ramp 1 to 8 secs___

3. Familiarize yourself with electrode placement site charts in your textbooks or recommended readings.

215

Orientation to Types of Electrode Placement Sites

1. There are numerous areas on the skin that exhibit decreased resistance to the flow of electrical current. What are the differences among them?

Motor Points: ___Are the anatomic location where the peripheral nerve enter the muscle.___

Trigger Points: ___Are those areas that exhibit hyper-sensitivity to both pressure and e-stim.___

Acupuncture Points: ___Another type of point that has been described for use w/ electrical stimulation devices___

page 8 Dermatomes: ___Areas of skin that are innervated by a particular nerve root are dermatomes___

10&11 Spinal Nerve Roots: ___Segmental levels___

2. What are some options for electrode placement sites if the patient had been referred to the department for pain management for the lower back?

Accupunture points for sensory analgesia

Observing Patient Responses to Electrode Placement Site Selections

1. Select one of your classmates to act as a patient to receive TENS application for pain management for his or her lower back. Position the patient so that the lower back is exposed and accessible and the patient is comfortable.

2. Prepare the electrodes and the unit to be applied to the patient.

Vertical Placement (Fig. 12-1)

1. Apply one channel of electrodes to the right side and one channel to the left side of the paraspinal musculature using the sites that you identified from the charts.

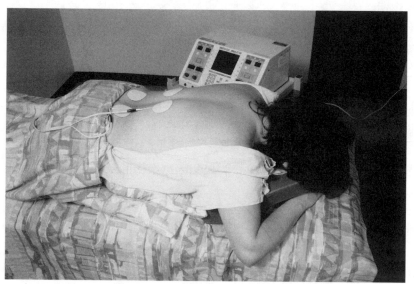

Figure 12-1 Two channels of electrodes set up with vertical electrode placements over the paraspinal muscles. A clinical stimulator is depicted; however, a portable device could also have been selected for this exercise.

2. Preset the parameters for sensory analgesia (ie, frequency, 70–120 Hz; pulse duration, 50 μsec). Slowly increase the intensity of the first channel and ask the patient to let you know when he or she first starts to feel something, where he or she feels it, and how it feels, and then to let you know when the intensity is strong but tolerable, and record these observations.

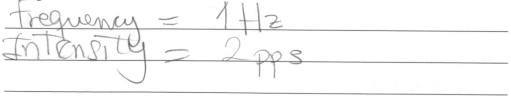

Frequency = 1 Hz

Intensity = 2 pps

3. Gradually increase the intensity of the second channel and repeat the sequence as above. Assess the area vertically between the electrodes. Were the intensity levels equal on both sides?

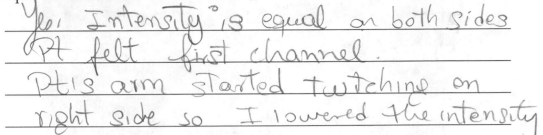

Yes, Intensity is equal on both sides. Pt felt first channel. Pt's arm started twitching on right side so I lowered the intensity

- What would explain this?

The intensity was set at the same rate and the left channel was turned on first & There was no pain felt by the patient

- Does the patient feel anything between the electrodes?

No

- What would explain this?

Because the channels are isolated on both paraspinal sides. Channels aren't crossing & were looking for a sensory response

4. Turn both intensities off. Leave the electrodes in place and disconnect the pin tips from the leads.

Horizontal Placement (Fig. 12-2)

1. Connect the leads to the electrodes so that there is one channel above L4-5 and one channel below. Repeat the same steps as above.

2. Preset the parameters for sensory analgesia (ie, frequency, 70–120 Hz; pulse duration, 50 μsec). Slowly increase the intensity of the first channel and ask the patient to let you know when he or she first starts to feel something, where he or she feels it, and how it feels, and then to let you know when the intensity is strong but tolerable, and record these observations.

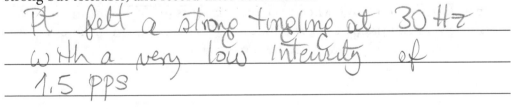

Pt felt a strong tingling at 30 Hz with a very low intensity of 1.5 PPS

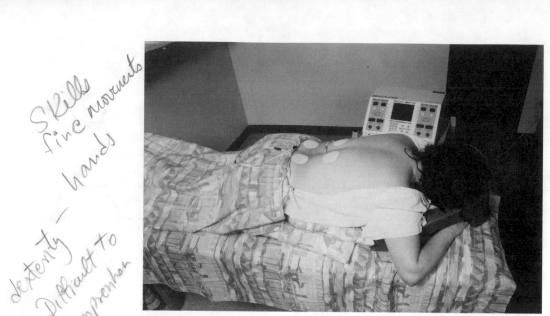

Figure 12-2 Two channels of electrodes set up with horizontal electrode placements above and below the area of discomfort. The electrodes are placed on paraspinal muscles but not on unilateral muscles.

3. Gradually increase the intensity of the second channel and repeat the sequence as above. Assess the area horizontally between the electrodes. Were the intensity levels equal on both sides?

   Frequency 1Hz
   Intensity - 1.5 pps It is the rate in which
   pt could tolerate stim before a muscle
   contraction was elicited

   • What would explain this?

   She was getting a strong enough stimulus
   To elicit a muscle contraction.

   • Does the patient feel anything between the electrodes?

   No

   • What would explain this?

   Because we are looking for sensory

4. Turn both intensities off. Leave the electrodes in place and disconnect the pin tips from the leads.

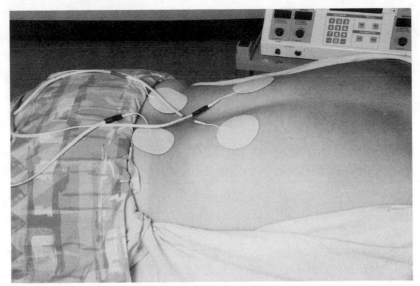

Figure 12-3 Two channels of electrodes set up with crossed electrode placements over the paraspinal muscles.

Criss-Cross Placement (Fig. 12-3)

1. Connect the leads to the electrodes so that one channel crosses the other channel.

2. Preset the parameters for sensory analgesia (ie, frequency, 70–120 Hz; pulse duration, 50 μsec). Slowly increase the intensity of the first channel and ask the patient to let you know when he or she first starts to feel something, where he or she feels it, and how it feels, and then to let you know when the intensity is strong but tolerable, and record these observations.

   Frequency = 1 Hz
   Intensity = 1 Pulse Rate
   Pt feels stronger response in lower right channel, could be because the area is more moist.

3. Gradually increase the intensity of the second channel and repeat the sequence as above. Assess the area between the electrodes. Were the intensity levels equal on both sides?

   Frequency = 1 Hz
   Intensity = .5 P.R.
   No they were not equal on both sides

- Was it easy for the patient to describe where he or she felt the sensation?

   Yes, Pt was able to give us a response as to where she felt the strongest sensation.

- What would explain this?

Could be because one area was more moist; pt doesn't have pain

- Does the patient feel anything between the electrodes?

Yes

- What would explain this?

Because the channels are crossing between one another

4. Did any of the set-ups produce more sensory stimulation than the others? Why or why not?

Criss-cross covering a layer surface are & the channels are crossed.

■ PROBLEM-SOLVING ACTIVITIES

Intensity Adjustment and Patient Instructions for Sensory Analgesia

1. Select one of your classmates to act as the patient and have TENS applied with a portable unit to his or her shoulder. Select electrode placement sites that encompass the entire shoulder and provide sensory analgesia throughout the local area.

2. Set up the electrodes as depicted in Figures 12-4 and 12-5. These represent GB 21 and LI 14 for one channel and SI 10 and SP 20 for the other channel. Why do you think these electrode placement sites were suggested, particularly in this crossed pattern?

Criss-crossed pattern gives the widest area of stimulation and possible pain relieve

3. Preset the parameters on the unit for sensory analgesia. Instruct the patient how and what to adjust to increase the intensity of the stimulation. Also instruct the patient in how and where to apply the electrodes, replace the battery, care for the portable TENS unit and electrodes, self-assess his or her level of discomfort, and record his or her assessment.

Textbook 227 page

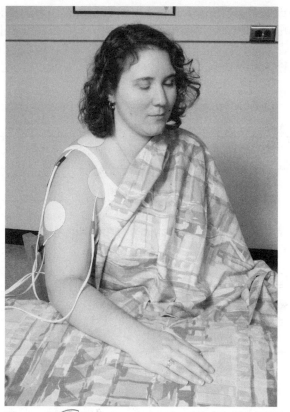

Figure 12-4 Anterior electrode placement sites for the shoulder.

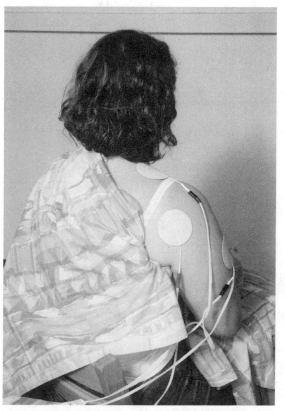

Figure 12-5 Posterior electrode placement sites for the shoulder.

4. Give the patient the TENS unit and ask him or her to increase the intensity to a strong but comfortable level. Instruct him or her to increase the intensity if the sensation "fades" at all. How did the setting of the intensity differ when the patient adjusted it?

1Hz and 1 pps was adequate stimulation for the pt. Pt had some difficulty placing electrodes on skin

5. What would be a possible rationale for instructing a patient how to adjust and care for a TENS unit?

To go over the important information concerning to safety and proper care of the TENS unit. Answer the pt's doubts and concerns about the TENS.

6. What additional considerations could there be for unit selection for a patient so that he or she could adjust the intensity? (dexterity, cognition)

Pt needs sufficient joint ROM & dexterity to apply electrodes, to plug in wires, and to operate the controls. Pt should have ability to understand the appropriate use of the machine

7. Would you expect the intensity for sensory analgesia to change while it was on? Why or why not?

No, because we want a sensory response no a muscle contraction, we want a strong, but comfortable tingling sensation.

8. What would happen if you increased the pulse duration of the stimulation?

Comfort decreases as phase duration increases

9. Would this ever be indicated? Why or why not?

Yes, Effective, carryover of pain relief is brief, because once the stimulation is turned off, normal sensation returns very rapidly

10. Instruct the patient how to terminate treatment, reassess, and remove his or her electrodes. What instructions did you find most difficult to explain to the patient?

To turn off the intensity before turn off the machine.

Applying and Observing Patient Response to Low Rate Stimulation for Analgesia for Low Back Pain

1. Select one of your classmates to receive application of motor level stimulation to his or her triceps surae bilaterally. One of the methods to help accomplish long-lasting pain relief is mediated by the release of endogenous opiates from the anterior pituitary deep within the brain. This is facilitated by at least 20 minutes of rhythmic muscle twitching. Selection of muscle groups that are segmentally related to the origin of the discomfort yet distal to the site tend to yield favorable patient responses.

2. Position the patient so that he or she is comfortable and supported with the ankles free to plantarflex and dorsiflex. Consult charts in your books to determine electrode placement sites and apply the electrodes to elicit a motor response from the triceps surae. Preset the TENS unit for motor level stimulation at a low rate.

3. Gradually increase the intensity until a twitch response is visible. Increase the intensity to the highest tolerable level so that joint movement is visible.

4. What are the differences between this level of stimulation and sensory analgesia?

Stimulation — twitching you see it

Sensory — is tingling you feel it

5. How long should it take for a patient to report some decrease in his or her discomfort following this mode of stimulation?

Ahmost immediate

6. What are the patient's subjective responses to this mode of stimulation?

Can no longer feel pain & the hand where the electrodes are feels colder than the other hand.

7. Under what circumstances might this mode be considered appropriate for a patient?

With pain and/or limited range of motion

8. What is the mechanism for pain relief that this mode is intended to induce?

Gate mechanism — blocks ascending pain.

9. Do you expect the patient to adapt to this mode of stimulation? Why or why not?

Yes. Due to acommodation

10. How long is the carry-over time for relief expected to be for this mode of stimulation?

There is potential for long-term carry over of pain relief

11. What possible rationale would there be for distally placed electrodes if this set-up was recommended for lower back pain?

Pts usually have a good response to choosing muscles segmentally related to the site of the discomfort but also distal to the site

Experiencing Noxious-Level Stimulation for Analgesia

1. Familiarize yourself with the stimulator. It must be capable of producing pulse durations in excess of 1 millisecond (1 msec). Select one of your classmates to be the patient for hyperstimulation to the web space of the back of his or her hand. Position the patient comfortably and position yourself so that you are at eye level with the patient.

2. There is probably a resistance meter of some form on the stimulator. It may measure conductance or resistance. Familiarize yourself with it by touching the two ends of the leads together and noting what the meter reads. Then hold the larger electrode in your hand and touch yourself with the probe electrode.

3. Compare the meter reading to your first reading. If it was lower, then the meter is reading conductance. If the second meter reading was higher, then it was reading resistance.

4. Preset the following parameters.

   - Frequency: 4 Hz
   - Pulse Duration: At least 1 msec
   - On Time: 30 sec per activation

5. Give the patient the dispersive/inactive electrode to hold in his or her other hand. You will not need gel or a conductive interface because the patient will grasp the electrode in the palm of his or her hand, which usually perspires when grasping something rubber. The perspiration will serve as the contact medium. Patients also tend to perspire when they are told that what they are going to experience will be a sensation similar to a hot needle or bee sting.

6. Locate the area that is most electrically active within the back of the web space of the back of the patient's hand. This would be the most conductive area (ie, HoKu or LI 4). Once it has been identified, press the on button and gradually increase the intensity while watching the patient's eyes. Your observation of the patient's eyes should let you know when the stimulus is as strong as he or she can tolerate. At that point, re-start the timer for 30 seconds. It is intended to be noxious. After the 30-second period is up, remove the probe and ask the patient to describe what he or she felt. Repeat for all members of your group.

7. When would noxious-level stimulation be indicated?

To stimule / activate the smaller pain fibers
A delta provide fast pain & C fibers deeper dull achy pain.

2 16

8. What would you need to explain to the patient to ensure that your chances of having it work would be enhanced?

You need to explain that it will painful but it will diminish the pain for 15 minutes after the accommodation

9. What possible explanations are there for positioning yourself at eye level with the patient?

Facial non verbal cues

10. Why would this type of stimulator have a conductance/resistance meter?

So we can measure the stimulater and resistance at the noxious level

11. How did the sensation of the stimulus differ from sensory analgesia?

There is a motor response in the stimulus and the sensory analgesia is more rapidly than w/ the sensory response.

IFC Electrode Placement Sites and Target Treatment Areas

1. IFC requires the use of two separate generators that produce a frequency greater than 100 Hz. The devices produce 2000 Hz, 4000 Hz, or 5000 Hz, which is referred to as the carrier frequency of the stimulator. Familiarize yourself with the parameters that are available and how you would adjust them.

2. What is the carrier frequency of the device that you are using?

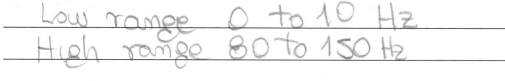
Dynatron 850 plus High range 80 to 150Hz
low range 0 to 10Hz

3. Are there any other carrier frequencies available on the device that you are using? If so, what are they?

Low range   0 to 10 Hz
High range 80 to 150 Hz

4. What would be the appropriate pulse burst rate, or beat frequency, for sensory analgesia?

> 50 beats per second

5. What would be the appropriate pulse burst rate, or beat frequency, for a tetanic motor response?

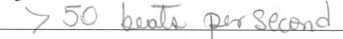
30 - 50 beats per second

Experiencing Interferential Electrical Stimulation and Movement of the Summation Field

Special Considerations With Interferential Electrical Stimulation Devices
- Interferential has the ability to pass through conductive tissues and summate; therefore, it must not be applied transthoracically, because the heart is a muscle.

1. Select a classmate to receive electrical stimulation to the knee. You will be applying IFC for generalized pain reduction throughout the knee joint, as if the patient had been diagnosed with chondromalacia of the patella that was producing pain posterior to the patella and inflammation on the superior medial aspect of the knee joint.

2. Position the patient so that the knee is supported in about 20 degrees of knee flexion (Fig. 12-6). Set up four electrodes of equal size so that the criss-cross is over the knee on both the medial and the lateral aspects of the knee (Fig. 12-7).

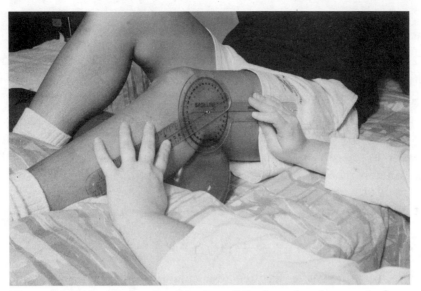

Figure 12-6 Appropriate positioning of the knee for placement of electrodes for treatment with IFC. The knee is supported and in an open joint position. (flexion)

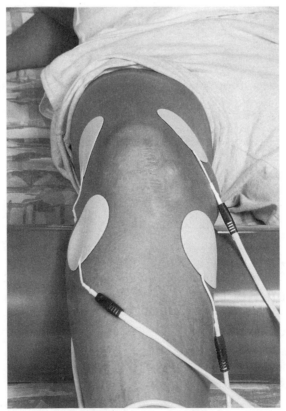

Figure 12-7 Knee with IFC applied using two channels of electrodes that have been crossed.

IFC mode for Pain

3. Slowly increase the intensity controls on both channels, and ask the patient to describe what he or she is feeling and where he or she is feeling it.

   8 mA lower lateral aspect of knee (lower electrodes
   11 mA until the patient can tolerate

4. What happens to the sensation when the patient increases knee flexion to about 90 degrees?

   It feels in the center the current once she got comfortable, but she first felt in the upper two electrodes once the intensity increase

5. Does the patient still feel the sensation in the same area?

   Yes

6. Can the patient tolerate more intensity now? If yes, increase the intensity. 12Hz

   she tolerated the most at

7. Locate the control on the device that will make the current move and ask the patient to describe what he or she feels. This control may be labeled "Dynamic," "Vector," or "Sweep."

   The pt felt the current move when the clinitian "swept" her finger over the target pad

8. Is it easier or more difficult for the patient to locate the stimulus than it was before you added the dynamic component to the IFC? Why or why not?

   It is easier because the current is more centralized

PATIENT SCENARIOS

Read through the patient scenarios and determine the following for each:

- Whether or not electrical stimulation would be indicated for pain relief
- What precautions there might be for the patient described
- What the parameter would be for the patient and your rationale for those parameters
- Where the electrodes should be placed, how many, and why
- Whether more than one mode could be indicated for pain relief
- Whether or not the patient might benefit from home use of a portable stimulator, and your rationale

A. Frank has been referred to the department for pain management. He has been diagnosed with herpes zoster, and on examination there is a large inflamed area on his left side. It starts in the thoracic region in midline posteriorly and extends anteriorly, tracing the last five ribs to the sternum. He is 85 years old, lives alone, and is otherwise healthy aside from an ulcer which has been controlled successfully by diet and medication for more than 20 years. His primary complaints are hypersensitivity to light touch throughout the inflamed area. It is so sensitive that he guards the area by flexing his trunk so that his clothing does not touch his skin on the left side.

B. Steve is a maintenance engineer for a retirement community. He has been referred to physical therapy for pain management subsequent to a low back injury he suffered while at work. He is a 42-year-old "workaholic" who has been performing strengthening exercises to stabilize his back. He has also worked through a "work-hardening program," and he is exceedingly anxious to return to his job. His only limitation is chronic low back pain. He is an avid bicyclist, canoeist, and hiker. He is looking for relief that will not interfere with his work with lawnmowers, power tools, and mechanical equipment.

C. Carol is a cartoonist who has been referred to physical therapy for pain management techniques subsequent to a cervical strain injury. She was involved in a motor vehicle accident where she was hit from behind. She now has muscle guarding and marked decreases in her cervical ROM in all directions. Her primary complaint is occipital headaches. She lives alone and works from a home office. Most of her day is spent at an artist's table, which is angled at 45 degrees. Medications to reduce muscle guarding and inflammation caused other complications with medications she was taking for depression.

DOCUMENTATION

Electrical stimulation can be used to control or reduce discomfort. Because there are a variety of ways in which this could be accomplished, it is important to document exactly what techniques produced favorable results for a patient. The following parameters must be documented:

- Treatment goal: Sensory analgesia or pain management
- Pretreatment pain assessment: Visual analog or other quantifiable measure
- Post-treatment pain assessment: Same instrument that was applied pretreatment

- Electrode placement sites: Documentation of exact electrode placement sites is not critical if the treatment goal is pain relief and the mode of stimulation is sensory analgesia. However, it can be helpful to the next clinician who treats the patient if alternate sites were used to help eliminate trial and error to achieve a successful result. Additionally, if an alternate mode of stimulation (e.g., hyperstimulation, low rate) was used to accomplish the treatment goal, then the stimulation sites must be documented.
- Specific stimulator used: If the mode of stimulation was sensory analgesia and it was accomplished with a clinical stimulator, then this is not critical to document. However, if the treatment involved home use of a TENS unit, the documentation should include the manufacturer and model of the device.

▰ LAB QUESTIONS

1. What was the most comfortable mode of stimulation for the patients?
2. What was the most uncomfortable mode of stimulation?
3. Which of the parameters would have accomplished A beta fiber stimulation?
4. What would the necessary parameters be for C fiber stimulation, and when might this be indicated?
5. The patient has increased the intensity to the highest level for a portable TENS unit, and they still do not feel the stimulation. What are the possible remedies, which would you employ first, and why?
6. Discuss TENS as a treatment technique in terms of the potential success rate as the sole treatment technique used to treat a patient.
7. Discuss the similarities and differences among the various electrode placement site selection options and provide the rationale for each.

Physical Agents for Transdermal Drug Delivery: Iontophoresis and Phonophoresis

13

This lab activity is designed to familiarize the student/learner with two potential application techniques for pushing medications through the skin: iontophoresis, in which ions are pushed through the skin, and phonophoresis, in which molecules are pushed through the skin.

Throughout this lab activity, student/learners are instructed to apply or experience different forms of phoresis commonly used in the clinic. Questions accompany each of the exercises. These questions are intended to help the student/learner learn how to incorporate the use of either iontophoresis or phonophoresis in clinical practice for the accomplishment of clinical treatment goals.

Part I: Iontophoresis

PURPOSE

This section focuses on the application of direct current for iontophoresis, which is the process of pushing like ions of something through the skin using an electrical charge of the same polarity. Student/learners will have the opportunity to phorese tap water through the skin with an iontophoresis device, including setting up the electrodes, setting the intensity, recording the tolerated intensity, and noting changes that may occur.

OBJECTIVES

Following the completion of this lab activity, the student/learner will be able to:

- Describe the components of an iontophoretic electrical stimulation device
- Describe the difference between the electrodes for iontophoresis and other forms of electrical stimulation
- Differentiate between the active and dispersive electrodes with an iontophoresis electrical stimulation device, and describe the rationale for why there is a large size difference between the two electrodes
- Apply iontophoresis to a classmate
- Determine the polarity of the active electrode with an iontophoretic electrical stimulation device
- Prepare the skin for the application of iontophoresis and predict common skin reactions that follow the application of iontophoresis
- Calculate dosage with iontophoresis using common techniques

EQUIPMENT THAT YOU WILL NEED
iontophoresis unit (electrodes, lead wires, and accessories)
moisturizing lotion

PRECAUTIONS AND WHY

Precaution	Why?
Decreased sensation	If the application involves the transmission of ions through the skin, the patient must be able to report sensation to avoid an adverse response.
Impaired cognitive ability	If the application involves the transmission of ions through the skin, the patient must be able to report sensation to avoid an adverse response.
Pregnancy	If the application is after the first trimester, there is little risk to the fetus or the patient. Electrical stimulation has been safely used for analgesia during labor and delivery, but it may interfere with fetal monitors.
Documented evidence of epilepsy, cerebral vascular accident, or reversible ischemic neurologic deficit	Patients should be monitored carefully when electrical stimulation is used in the cervical region. Possible adverse responses may include temporary change in cognitive status, headache, vertigo, and other neurological signs.

CONTRAINDICATIONS AND WHY

Contraindication	Why?
Pregnancy (first trimester)	There is no data to indicate the level of safety for the fetus with the application of electrical stimulation during the first trimester of pregnancy.
Over the carotid sinus	If the circulation to the brain is altered, there could be adverse effects.
Pacemaker	Electrical stimulation devices may interfere with the electrical demands of the pacemaker.
Cancerous lesions	Most application techniques have the potential to produce an increase in circulation to the area. The possibility exists that electrical stimulation over or in proximity to cancerous lesions may enhance the development of metastasis.
Known allergy to the prescribed medication	Iontophoresis involves pushing the medication through the skin to be picked up by the bloodstream. If the patient is allergic to the medication, serious complications could result.

LAB ACTIVITIES

Orientation to the Equipment

Iontophoresis involves pushing ions through the skin. After a patient receives a physician's prescription for the medication, the medication-saturated electrode, which is polar, is carefully applied to the same pole of the electrical stimulator, causing the ions to be repelled into the patient. Direct low level current then can be applied to repel the medication's ions into the bloodstream below the surface of the skin.

1. What parameters do you see on the direct current device?

    _____

    _____

    _____

    _____

2. What parameters are not available on this device that were available for your use to accomplish motor levels of stimulation?

    _____

    _____

    _____

    _____

3. What accessories for the direct current device are available?

    _____

    _____

    _____

    _____

4. How many channels does this stimulator have?

    _____

    _____

    _____

    _____

5. Why does this device differ from the stimulators that you have previously used for motor levels of electrical stimulation?

    _____

    _____

    _____

    _____

Determination of Dosage with Iontophoresis

Dosage for iontophoresis is not based on patient sensation. This is a different type of electrical stimulation that does not rely on a motor level of response or a sensory level of stimulation. Most often, the patient will report that there is no sensation during the application of direct current. Dosage is most commonly related to a formula that includes time and intensity.

Common Application Techniques

$$\text{intensity} \times \text{treatment time} = 40$$
$$\text{mAmps} \times \text{minutes} = \text{mAmp minutes}$$

mAmp		Minutes		Dosage
1	×	40	=	40 mAmp min
2	×	20	=	40 mAmp min
4	×	10	=	40 mAmp min

The longer that the stimulation is left on, the lower the intensity can be. This decreases the potential adverse effects from the current itself.

Cautions With Direct Current Applications

- Always ask the patient whether or not he or she is allergic to the medication that will be applied during the iontophoresis treatment. It is the responsibility of the clinician to document that the patient has stated that there is no known allergy to the medication to be administered before treatment begins.
- Direct current may cause an itching sensation underneath the electrode. This may be a sign of tissue burning. Patients should be cautioned to call the clinician if this occurs during the treatment.
- Patients must be cautioned not to touch or move the electrodes during the treatment time with direct current. This could affect current density and potentially result in a burn.

Phoresing Tap Water

1. Select a classmate/patient to have tap water phoresed into his or her forearm and anatomical snuff box. Inspect the skin in the treatment area and make sure that it is clean, free of oils and/or surface debris. Some units recommend that the areas under both electrodes be scrubbed with soap and water before the application of iontophoresis. The scrubbing helps to further reduce skin resistance, which enhances the flow of current across the skin.

2. Read the instructions for filling the electrodes for the iontophoresis unit that you are using, and prepare both the active and dispersive electrodes. For this activity, both electrodes will be prepared with tap water.

3. Apply the active electrode to the anatomical snuff box (Fig. 13-1). When treating an actual patient, the active electrode must be the same polarity as the medication.

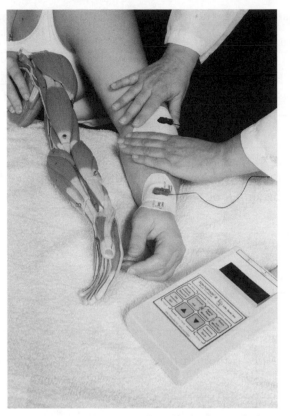

Figure 13-1 The active (smaller) electrode is placed over the anatomical snuff box and the dispersive (larger) electrode is placed over the proximal extent of the extensor muscle belly.

4. Apply the dispersive electrode to the muscle belly of the wrist extensors approximately 3 inches from the active electrode. The dispersive electrode is larger (usually at least 2 times) than the active electrode and is placed over muscle, an electrically conductive area which has low resistance.

5. Turn the unit on and slowly increase the intensity using the dosage chart. Try each of the intensity levels to see what it feels like. Remember that it is better if the patient does not feel anything. Longer treatment times permit transdermal passage of the medication across the skin with less skin irritation. Intensity should not exceed 1 mAmp/cm^2 of the active surface area of the electrode to avoid tissue burn due to concentration of energy.

6. Record your settings:

    Intensity (mAmp): _____

    Minutes: _____

    Dosage: _____

7. What sensations does the patient report at the settings that you selected?

_____

_____

_____

_____

8. When the treatment time ends, turn the intensity off and remove the electrodes. How does the skin look?

_____

_____

_____

_____

9. How did the area underneath the electrodes feel to the patient?

_____

_____

_____

_____

10. It is quite common to find etching and erythema under both electrodes. It is recommended that clinicians apply a moisturizer to the area following treatment with iontophoresis.

11. What, if anything, did you learn from your application of iontophoresis that you can use with patients in future applications?

_____

_____

_____

_____

LAB QUESTIONS

1. Why didn't the iontophoresis unit have a frequency control or a pulse duration control?
2. What would happen if an electrode fell off during treatment? What would the patient feel?

Part II: Phonophoresis

PURPOSE

Phonophoresis is a technique that uses ultrasound to deliver medication through the skin. Clinical research has yet to provide unequivocal support for the use of ultrasound as a mode of delivery for medication; however, techniques to ensure that the acoustical conductivity of medications specifically prepared for phonophoresis are presented. Student/learners will test ultrasound transducers and medications to determine the acoustical conductivity of the medications and potential for being pushed through the skin.

OBJECTIVES

Following the completion of this lab activity, the student/learner will be able to:

- Test an ultrasound transducer using water to determine whether there is acoustical output
- Test medications used for phonophoresis to determine whether there is acoustical conductivity sufficient to pass through the medication and push it through the skin

EQUIPMENT THAT YOU WILL NEED:

variable-frequency ultrasound unit (1 MHz, 3 MHz)   towels
pillows   cup of water
ultrasound gel (acoustically conductive gel)   cellophane tape
medication to be tested for acoustical conductivity   cotton-tipped applicator

PRECAUTIONS AND WHY

Precaution	Why?
Open wounds	Sterile saline must fill the wound for transmission of the acoustical energy.
Impaired cognitive ability	The patient must be able to communicate any uncomfortable sensation under the transducer.
Pregnancy	During the later stages of pregnancy there is no data to indicate that there would be any adverse effects as long as the treatment area does not include the abdomen, ankle,* or lower back (1 MHz).

Precaution	Why?
Peripheral vascular disease	The presence of peripheral vascular disease is not a problem in itself; however, if the treatment area is involved, the patient's tissues may not be able to maintain homeostasis or respond to an increase in tissue temperature.
Advanced age	As long as the patient is alert and their sensation is intact, ultrasound should not cause any difficulties.
Previous experience with ultrasound	The patient may or may not have had a positive experience. It is important to elicit this from the patient, in addition to explaining the rationale for *this* application for *this* diagnosis.
Over joint or metal implants	Ultrasound may cause heterogenous heating within the joint if a cementing media was used. To avoid this, use 3 MHz ultrasound, which does not have sufficient depth to reach the internal aspects of joints. Metal implants tend to elevate in temperature faster than bone, but they also dissipate the heat faster, making them safe for ultrasound application.
Pain with pressure	Ultrasound involves the movement of a transducer along the surface of the skin. If this type of pressure is painful for a patient, an underwater technique with ultrasound can be employed.

*There is an accupuncture point located on the medial aspect of the ankle that may be highly active and potentially dangerous if stimulated during pregnancy.

■ CONTRAINDICATIONS AND WHY

Contraindication	Why?
Known allergy to the prescribed medication	Phonophoresis involves pushing the medication through the skin to be picked up by the bloodstream. If the patient is allergic to the medication, serious complications could result.
Pregnancy	There is no physical therapy indication for application of ultrasound over a pregnant uterus, and there is no data to indicate what effect, if any, the therapeutic application of ultrasound would have on a fetus.
Abnormal growth (presumed malignant)	Thermal applications of ultrasound can potentially elevate tissue temperature, increase circulation to the area, and thus may enhance the growth.
Metastasis	Thermal applications of ultrasound can potentially elevate tissue temperature, increase circulation to the area, and thus may enhance the growth or spread malignancy to other tissues.
Lack of sensation (thermal application)	If the patient is unable to report pain, they can easily burn with thermal applications of ultrasound.

Contraindication	Why?
Thrombus	The application of ultrasound directly over a thrombus may cause the clot to dislodge and move to the heart, lungs, or brain.
Pacemaker	There is no indication to apply ultrasound directly over a pacemaker. The potential for interference between the pacemaker and the ultrasound device exists.
Psoriasis	Ultrasound must be applied to the skin via an acoustical media without airspace. Psoriatic skin may have too many irregularities to permit passage of the ultrasound into the patient.

▪ LAB ACTIVITIES

Testing the Transducer for Acoustical Output

1. Select a transducer that is waterproof.

2. Apply a small amount of the medication to be tested to the surface of the transducer using a cotton-tipped applicator, making sure to cover the surface of the transducer.

3. Make a ring of cellophane tape around the transducer so that you are creating a "well" that can be filled with water (Fig. 13-2).

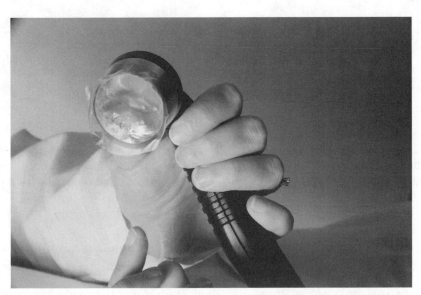

Figure 13-2 Cellophane tape ring around the surface of the ultrasound transducer.

4. Pour some tap water into the well so that the water depth is about ¼ inch (Fig. 13-3).

5. Set the following parameters: 1 MHz, 1.5 W/cm².

6. Look at the transducer surface. If there is a disturbance in the water, then there is acoustical output from the transducer (Fig. 13-4). If there is no disturbance in the surface of the water, this means one of two things.

   • There is no acoustical output from the ultrasound device

   OR

   • The medication is not acoustically conductive, which means that the medication will not be transmitted through the skin using phonophoresis

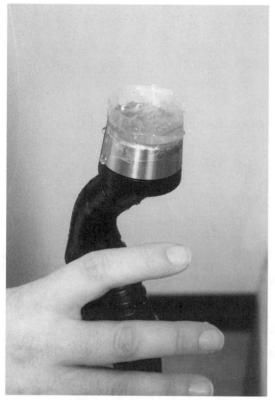

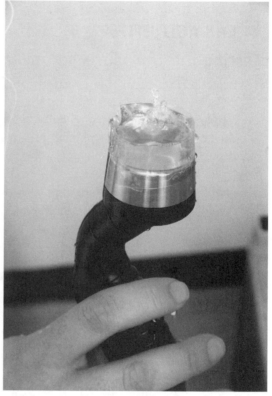

Figure 13-3 Approximately ¼ inch of tap water is added to the top of the transducer to fill the "well" that has been created with the cellophane tape.

Figure 13-4 Acoustical energy being transmitted through the well of water on a transducer that has been coated with a medication indicates that the medication does in fact conduct acoustical energy.

7. To determine whether there is acoustical output from the ultrasound device, clean the medication from the transducer surface and then repeat the above steps.

   • If the surface of the water is disturbed, then it was the medication that impeded the transmission of the ultrasound.
   • If the surface of the water is not disturbed, then the ultrasound transducer requires repair, because it is not producing acoustical energy.

8. Repeat the process with another ultrasound transducer and the same medication to determine whether or not the medication is acoustically conductive.

This process of testing the medication and the transducer is a good technique to periodically employ to determine whether the transducer is producing ultrasound, especially because it is common for the patient not to feel anything during the application of ultrasound. Weekly checks of the acoustical output of ultrasound transducers are beneficial for clinicians to help assure that there is in fact acoustical energy being emitted from the transducer.

◼ LAB QUESTIONS

1. How would treatment time with phonophoresis change, if at all, if the medication you were instructed to apply was prescribed for acute inflammation?
2. What additional precautions would there be for the application of phonophoresis that you did not have for the application of ultrasound? Why?
3. How would you be able to determine whether the patient had an adverse response to the ultrasound or to the medication administered following a treatment with phonophoresis?
4. Why was it suggested that the medication be applied to the surface of the transducer and then water applied on top of that to test the conductivity of the medication?
5. If you were instructed to apply phonophoresis to a patient, would you need to use any lotion or gel in addition to the medication? Why or why not?

Integration of Physical Agents: Clinical Decision Making

14

Tools for any task are only as useful as their user. In other words, you may have excellent tools, but they are useless if you do not know how to use them. This lab activity has deliberately been placed last in this manual. You have been presented with many different therapeutic tools that can be used to accomplish the following common treatment goals.

- Acute pain reduction
- Chronic pain reduction
- Muscle guarding reduction
- Muscle strengthening
- Muscle atrophy prevention
- Edema reduction via muscle pump
- Tissue healing
- Relieving pressure on nerve roots to help reduce paresthesias

The first part of this lab activity focuses on the electrical stimulation devices themselves as tools to accomplish therapeutic treatment goals. The second part requires the student/learner to compare physical agent modalities in terms of the potential benefits and the potential harm that may inadvertently be caused with the use of each.

Part I: Devices in Terms of Accomplishing Treatment Goals

◤ PURPOSE

Each of the previous lab activities that concerned electrical stimulation presented parameters to accomplish goals as a way of introducing you to the device. In this chapter, the focus is specifically on the goal and how to make the stimulator do what you want it to, or how to determine whether or not it is capable of doing what you want it to. Referring to previous laboratory exercises will be helpful.

◤ OBJECTIVES

Following the completion of this lab activity, the student/learner will be able to:

- Translate the terminology into the application parameters for electrical stimulation for the accomplishment of therapeutic treatment goals
- Interpret the information that is presented on a manufacturer's product specification sheet for electrical stimulation devices to determine what the product is capable of doing in a clinical environment
- Compare and contrast several different specification sheets of electrical stimulation devices to determine potential applications for therapeutic interventions
- Translate technical information into application techniques for therapeutic goal accomplishment

- Compare and contrast the treatment goals with the capability of described electrical stimulation devices
- Select treatment parameters based on treatment goals for a given stimulator

◼ EQUIPMENT THAT YOU WILL NEED

various electrical stimulation devices
electrodes and lead wires for each of the devices
product specification sheets for electrical stimulation devices
advertisements for electrical stimulation devices

◼ LAB ACTIVITIES

Treatment Goals and Electrical Stimulation Parameters

1. Treatment goals for electrical stimulation include pain reduction, edema reduction, muscle strengthening, muscle re-education, and the reduction of muscle guarding. Select one of the stimulators and identify which treatment goals could be accomplished with the device based on the parameters available for that device.

Device: _____

Treatment Goals	Parameters
Pain reduction	
Edema reduction	
Muscle strengthening	
Muscle re-education	
Reduction of muscle guarding	

2. Identify which treatment goals could not be accomplished using the stimulator that you selected. Why not?

_____

_____

_____

_____

3. Select another electrical stimulation device, and repeat the exercise.

Device: _____

Treatment Goals	Parameters
Pain reduction	
Edema reduction	
Muscle strengthening	
Muscle re-education	
Muscle spasm reduction	

4. Identify which treatment goals could not be accomplished using this stimulator. Why not?

_____

_____

_____

_____

5. What are the common parameters for an electrical stimulator to be able to produce a contraction in an innervated muscle?

_____

_____

_____

_____

6. What parameters are necessary for the unit to be able to accomplish edema reduction or muscle strengthening?

_____

_____

_____

_____

7. What are the necessary parameters for the unit to be able to accomplish sensory analgesia?

_____

_____

_____

_____

Comparing Devices and Applications

1. Review the mock specification sheets that follow.

Excellence in Stimulation	
Frequency:	0.1–1000 pps
Pulse duration:	50 μsec up to 2 sec
Intensity:	up to 1 mA
Channels:	2, 4, 6, or 8 independent channels
ON/OFF:	20-, 30-, 40-minute ON times
Ramps:	0.1 to 1 second up and down

Superb Stimulator	
Frequency:	pain, edema, spasm
Pulse duration:	comfortable
Intensity:	sufficient for excellent pain relief
Channels:	1 or 2
ON/OFF:	unit beeps three short times to indicate end of treatment
Ramps:	no uncomfortable surging

Sensational Stimulation	
Frequency:	1–250 pps (2500 Hz or 5000 Hz carrier frequency)
Pulse duration:	100–200 μsec (burst durations will vary)
Intensity:	up to 200 mA, 2 kω load tested
Channels:	1, 2, or 4 channels with independent current generators
ON/OFF:	4/4, 10/10, 10/50, or adjustable from continuous to independent times
Ramps:	independent ON/OFF ramps from 0.1 to 5 seconds

CREATIVE CURRENTS

Frequency:	1–120 pps
Pulse duration:	fixed at 50 μsec
Intensity:	1–500 volts
Channels:	1 bifurcated lead channel
Ramps:	not applicable
Waveform:	twin spike, no net DC, polarity adjustable ±

2. Indicate which treatment goals each of the devices are capable of performing.

Treatment Goals	Excellence	Superb	Sensational	Creative
Sensory analgesia				
Numbness				
Muscle strengthening				
Muscle spasm reduction				

3. What additional information, if any, would you need to make this determination?

_____

_____

_____

_____

4. Was any of the terminology used in the materials presented inappropriate or jargon? If so, which stimulators?

_____

_____

_____

_____

5. Was the information clear?

_____

_____

_____

_____

6. Would you be able to determine what the device could be used for if you were not able to speak with anyone about the device?

_____

_____

_____

_____

7. A salesman comes into the physical therapy department and presents an inservice program on a new stimulator. He claims that his stimulator can treat all symptoms at the same time. What is wrong with this statement?

_____

_____

_____

_____

■ PATIENT SCENARIOS

Select an electrical stimulation device from those described in the lab activity to accomplish the treatment goal for each of the following patients.

A. It is late in the afternoon, and several patients are being treated with electrical stimulation units whose specifications were provided in this lab activity. You are in search of a stimulator to accomplish reduction in muscle guarding. All of the units except the Creative Currents unit are already being used. What would be the most appropriate course of action for you to take?

B. Don, an Olympic pole-vaulter, is being treated in your clinic for a tear to his hamstrings. Which of the units described previously, if any, could be used for pain relief? Which of the units could be used for muscle pumping to increase the nutrients into the vastus medialis? Which of the units could be used for tissue healing?

C. Jane is an occupational therapist who is being treated in the physical therapy department for her painful, edematous ankles. She is now at the end of her second trimester carrying twins. What potential treatment options do you have for her (if any) with stimulators described previously?

D. Susan is an athletic trainer for the local community college women's field hockey team. She spends a great deal of time kneeling while taping the ankles of the team members. She fell down on her knees and has been diagnosed with chondromalacia of the patella in both knees. There is marked weakness of the vastus medialis, edema superior to the patella, and a palpable painful crepitus in both knees when descending stairs. The treatment goals include pain relief, edema reduction, and muscle strengthening. Of the four devices described previously, which would be useful for addressing which of the many treatment goals?

■ DOCUMENTATION

Select two of the classmates/patients to whom you applied modalities during the lab activities and write a progress note that includes each patient's subjective complaints, the objective information that you recorded, the physical agent that was applied, the manner of application, the response to the applied physical agent, and your assessment.

Part II: Clinical Decision Making With All Physical Agent Modalities

■ PURPOSE

This lab activity provides the student/learner with the opportunity to integrate everything he or she has learned from the previous lab activities and use that experience to apply clinical decision-making techniques in the clinical environment.

■ OBJECTIVES

Following the completion of this lab activity, the student/learner will be able to:

- Discriminate between physical agent modalities that can be used to accomplish similar treatment goals
- Develop a scenario where more than one modality may be used to accomplish a cumulative goal
- Scrutinize common practice techniques to determine potential benefits and risks to the patient

■ LAB ACTIVITIES

Cross-Referencing Treatment Goals With Therapeutic Interventions

1. Place a check next to all the possible physical agent modalities that could be used to treat the listed symptoms.

	Heat	Ice	US	DC	ES	Traction	CPM	Hydro	IC
Pain									
Muscle guarding									
Muscle weakness									
Tissue healing time									
Nerve root compression									
Spasticity									
Hyper-sensitivity									

	Heat	Ice	US	DC	ES	Traction	CPM	Hydro	IC
Edema									
Acute in-flammation									
Chronic in-flammation									
Hematoma									

CPM, continuous passive motion; DC, direct current; ES, electrical stimulation; IC, intermittent compression; US, ultrasound.

2. Place a check next to all the possible physical agent modalities that could be used to increase the listed goals.

	Heat	Ice	US	DC	ES	Traction	CPM	Hydro	IC
Motor control									
Muscle strength									
Range of motion (stretching)									
Muscle function									

3. Place a check next to the modalities that would be contraindicated if the patient was pregnant, by trimester.

	Heat	Ice	US	DC	ES	Traction	CPM	Hydro	IC
First trimester									
Second trimester									
Third trimester									

4. A patient has been diagnosed as having an acute cervical strain. She complains of pain, decreased ROM, muscle guarding, and tingling in the fingers of her right hand. What modalities could you potentially combine to treat this patient and accomplish the treatment goals?

_____

_____

_____

_____

5. Would ice or heat be indicated? Why?

_____

_____

_____

_____

6. Would there be a situation in which either heat or ice would be appropriate? If yes, when?

_____

_____

_____

_____

7. On consultation with a senior therapist, traction, ultrasound, and moist heat have been recommended to treat the patient. Which of the suggestions would you use?

_____

_____

_____

_____

8. If you decided to use more than one treatment modality, how would you sequence them? Why?

_____

_____

_____

_____

9. What positioning would be most appropriate for this patient? Why?

_____

_____

_____

_____

10. Patient education is an important part of any therapeutic intervention. What things must you keep in mind when instructing this patient?

_____

_____

_____

_____

11. What behaviors do you want to be sure to warn this patient against?

_____

_____

_____

_____

12. After applying all of the suggested modalities, the patient complained of a deep aching sensation in the cervical musculature. What might this indicate?

_____

_____

_____

_____

13. How would you protect against this in the future?

_____

_____

_____

_____

14. If, after treatment with traction, muscle guarding was no longer apparent and pain was reduced to a more tolerable level, would you proceed with ultrasound to the area as previously planned? Why or why not? (NOTE: Both answers are possible!)

_____

_____

_____

_____

15. If, after ultrasound, the patient reported that there was no paresthesia present, would you apply traction? Why or why not?

_____

_____

_____

_____

16. After treatment using any or all of the modalities mentioned the patient reported that he or she now had a throbbing headache. What could this indicate?

_____

_____

_____

_____

■ PATIENT SCENARIOS

A. Kenny is a weekend warrior who played rugby with college friends over the weekend. He has had his right knee replaced, his left ankle fused, his right hip pinned, and his rotator cuff repaired two times. Kenny does not seem to experience pain until real physical damage has occurred. He has been referred to therapy for an acute episode of torticollis that is producing marked muscle guarding in the right sternocleidomastoid. Once again, James reports no pain. He has commented that he actually has no sensation on the right sternocleidomastoid, it just "feels hard" when he touches it. A senior therapist in the department has recommended that you use heat and stretching to treat the torticollis.

- What are your plans? How would you explain them to Kenny and to the observing student?

_____

_____

_____

_____

B. Pete is an architect who has been referred to therapy for the relief of pain and muscle guarding in his lower back. He has difficulty maintaining an upright posture and has been told that he has a "lateral shift." On examination, Pete has weak abdominals and paraspinal muscle guarding in the lumbar and thoracic spinal musculature. He complains of pain down the right leg into his ankle and difficulty getting up from a supine position.

- What physical agent therapeutic modalities could potentially be used? Also state the goal, the parameters to accomplish the goal, and the sequence if you suggest more than one modality.

Modality	Goal	Parameters	Sequence

C. You are filling in at a local out-patient therapy clinic. On reading the patient notes you discover that all the patients that you are expected to see are to receive hot packs, ultrasound, and massage in addition to joint mobilization, therapeutic exercise, and ice.

- What are the potential patient treatment goals for which this scenario would be appropriate?

_____

_____

_____

_____

- How would you proceed in that setting with the circumstances as described?

_____

_____

_____

_____

D. After a biomedical engineering check of the ultrasound units in the clinic, it is determined that the ultrasound unit is no longer producing anything therapeutic. You recall using it yesterday, and having patients report that they felt better when you were finished with the ultrasound.

- What could potentially have caused these patients to feel better?

_____

_____

_____

_____

- How would you be able to avoid treating patients with an ultrasound device that isn't working properly in the future?

_____

_____

_____

_____

E. A patient is to receive the following therapeutic modalities: stretching exercises, ultrasound, and moist heat.

- Suggest a logical sequence for these interventions and provide your rationale.

_____

_____

_____

_____

F. You are observing a treatment in which electrodes are applied to the patient's elbow, and the therapist appears to be performing transverse friction massage to the lateral epicondyle.

- For what purpose is the therapist doing both manual techniques and electrical stimulation at the same time?

  _____

  _____

  _____

  _____

- What is the potential rationale for the electrical stimulation?

  _____

  _____

  _____

  _____

- What would the parameters need to be for this to potentially be beneficial for the patient?

  Placement: _____

  No. of Electrodes: _____

  Pulse Duration: _____

  Frequency/Beat: _____

  Intensity/Sensation: _____

- If you were then asked to apply ice while the electrical stimulation continued, would this be a good idea or poor idea in your opinion? Why?

  _____

  _____

  _____

  _____

  _____

Appendix:
Application Techniques
and Sequences

NEUROMUSCULAR ELECTRICAL STIMULATION

1. Review the precautions and contraindications before applying neuromuscular electrical stimulation (NMES) to ensure that this application is safe for this patient at this time.

2. Inspect the lead wires to ensure that they are intact and there are no breaks in the protective outer covering surrounding the wires.

3. Select electrodes that are appropriate for the application based on the size of the muscle in which you will be eliciting a contraction.

4. Explain the modality to the patient so that he or she will know what to expect from the application of NMES, which will cause his or her muscles contract.

5. Ask the patient to rate his or her discomfort on a scale of 1 to 10, with 1 representing no pain and 10 representing the worst pain possible. Record that number in the patient's chart.

6. Inspect the skin overlying the muscles to which the NMES will be applied. Assess for blanching, increased temperature, the presence of scars, and absent or altered sensation. If there are any irregularities not sufficient to cause a change in the treatment approach, note them in the patient's chart and continue with the application.

7. Remove the patient's clothing in the treatment area, making sure that proximal joints are not restricted.

8. Clean the skin before applying the electrodes, making sure that there are no lotions, oils, or anything else that might inhibit the uniform flow of electrical energy into the patient.

9. Prepare the electrodes for application to the patient according to the directions on the packaging. Moist electrode interfaces help to decrease the resistance to the flow of current and make the sensation more comfortable for the patient with less intensity.

10. Place one of your hands on the muscle belly from which you are attempting to elicit a response. Your other hand should resist the contraction. Ask the patient to contract against you. This should provide you with a palpable muscle contraction and the location of the center of the muscle belly, as long as the muscle is innervated and the patient has at least a 3/5 grade for muscle strength.

11. Place one of the electrodes over the center of the muscle belly and the other electrode distal on the muscle belly. Alternately, you can follow the electrode placement sites listed on motor point charts.

12. Position the patient so he or she is supported for the application of the NMES. Depending on the treatment goal and the muscles stimulated, you may restrain the distal portion of the extremity to provide resistance or ensure that the contraction is isometric. This will depend on treatment goals and patient diagnosis.

13. Apply the NMES electrodes to the patient making sure that there is good contact between the electrodes and the skin. It may be necessary to secure the electrodes with a strap to help conform them to the surface of the patient's affected body part.

14. Drape the patient so that no unnecessary skin is exposed.

15. Set the parameters according to the treatment goals and the level of disability of the patient.
    - Equal on and off times to start out a treatment program
    - Longer off times and shorter on times for weaker patients
    - Gradually increase the intensity of the contraction
    - Progress to 10 on and 50 off for maximum muscle strengthening with 10 contractions

16. Stay with the patient during the first one or two cycles to ensure that he or she understands what to expect from the stimulation cycles and contractions with NMES.

17. Provide the patient with a means to contact you during the treatment time if needed. Remind the patient what to expect from the NMES application and to let you know if it feels uncomfortable.

18. Re-check the patient after 3 to 5 minutes to ensure that he or she is still comfortable.

19. When the treatment time concludes, remove the electrodes from the patient and check the skin for signs of irritation. Note any abnormal responses in the patient's chart.

20. Explain to the patient what he or she potentially could expect later in the day as a result of the application of NMES, including how the stimulated muscles might feel and what to do if the muscles feel fatigued.

◼ TRACTION

1. Review the precautions and contraindications before applying traction to ensure that its use is safe for this patient at this time.

2. Explain the modality to the patient so that he or she will know what to expect from the application of traction.

3. Position the belts on the traction table so that when the patient lies down he or she will do so on top of the belts and will not have to move as much.

4. Ask the patient whether he or she needs to use the restroom before setting up the traction.

5. Position the patient for the application of the traction so that he or she is supported in a neutral position.
   • For treatment of the lumbar spine, the patient should be treated supine with a foot stool topped by a pillow under the knees to put the hips and knees in 90 degrees of flexion. (There are other positions, but this is the most common.)
   • Treatment of the cervical muscles should also take place with the patient supine with pillows for support to allow the postural muscles to be unloaded.

6. Check the patient to ensure that his or her alignment is straight from head to toe.

7. Set the parameters for the traction. Separation of the intervertebral segments occurs when the traction force is applied in a sufficient amount.
   • For lumbar traction, ask the patient how much he or she weighs and set the traction to approximately one fourth that amount.
   • For cervical traction, the amount of poundage starts at 10 lb.

8. Mechanical traction devices provide numerous options for pull and relax times. A minimum of 7 seconds of pull time is commonly administered to allow for separation to occur. An equal rest time is appropriate but can be adjusted based on patient comfort.

9. Provide the patient with a means to contact you during the treatment time if needed. Remind the patient what to expect from the traction application and to let you know if it feels uncomfortable.

10. Re-check the patient after 3 to 5 minutes to ensure that he or she is still comfortable.

11. When the treatment time concludes, turn off the traction unit and loosen the straps.

12. Allow the patient to rest in the unloaded position for a few minutes.

13. Remove the straps. Be careful to have the patient roll to one side to stand up rather than sit up. Do not have him or her sit on the edge of the table. (this would increase disc pressure)

14. Assess the outcome of the application of the traction and document your findings. Also document the parameters of the traction that was applied.

■ INTERMITTENT COMPRESSION DEVICES

1. Review the precautions and contraindications before applying intermittent compression devices to ensure that its use is safe for this patient at this time.

2. Explain the modality to the patient so that he or she will know what to expect from the application of intermittent compression devices.

3. Inspect the skin over the area where the intermittent compression device will be applied. Assess for blanching, increased temperature, and absent or altered sensation. If there are any irregularities not sufficient to cause a change in the treatment approach, note them in the patient's chart and continue with the application.

4. Measure the girth and or volume of the edematous extremity and record your findings on the chart for comparison with post-treatment measurements.

5. Monitor and record the patient's blood pressure and heart rate.

6. Ask the patient if he or she needs to use the restroom before the application of intermittent compression.

7. Position the patient for the application of intermittent compression so that the edematous extremity is supported in a neutral position but elevated above the heart. For example, if you were treating the upper extremity, the patient would be treated supine with the upper extremity elevated and supported with pillows.

8. Apply a stockinette to the extremity to maintain cleanliness and absorb any perspiration that may occur during the treatment time. Then apply the intermittent compression sleeve designed for that extremity to the patient. Attach the hoses to the appliance and the device.

9. Drape the patient so that no other skin is exposed.

10. Follow the instructions on the intermittent compression device regarding the set up of the device. Select the appropriate inflation/deflation pressures. Ensure that the inflation pressure is less than the patient's systolic blood pressure.

11. Provide the patient with a means to contact you during the treatment time if needed. Remind the patient what to expect from the intermittent compression device application and to let you know if it feels uncomfortable.

12. Re-check the patient after 10 to 15 minutes to ensure that he or she is still comfortable.

13. When the treatment time concludes, remove the extremity from the appliance and check the area that was treated. Inspect the skin for normal and abnormal physiological responses. Note any abnormal responses in the patient's chart.

14. Measure the girth and or volume of the treated extremity and record your findings for comparison with pretreatment findings.

15. Ask the patient for any subjective responses to the treatment and record his or her comments.

■ IONTOPHORESIS

1. Review the precautions and contraindications before applying iontophoresis to ensure that its use is safe for this patient at this time.

2. Inspect the lead wires to ensure that they are intact and there are no breaks in the protective outer covering surrounding the wires.

3. Explain the modality to the patient so that he or she will know what to expect from the application of iontophoresis.

4. Ask the patient whether he or she has an allergy to the medication that has been prescribed for the iontophoresis. Document the patient's response to your question. If the patient is allergic to the medication, contact the prescribing physician for an alternative medication. Do not continue with treatment.

5. Inspect the skin overlying the treatment area where iontophoresis will be applied. Assess for blanching, increased temperature, the presence of scars, and absent or altered sensation. If there are any irregularities not sufficient to cause a change in the treatment approach, note them in the patient's chart and continue with the application.

6. Remove the patient's clothing in the treatment area and ensure adequate access.

7. Clean the skin before applying the electrodes, making sure that there are no lotions, oils, or anything else that might inhibit the uniform flow of electrical energy into the patient.

8. Review the medication to determine its polarity. The medication must be applied to the electrode of the same polarity.

9. Prepare the electrodes for application to the patient according to the directions on the packaging. Ensure that the medicated electrode is saturated with the medication.

10. Apply the medicated electrode to the target treatment area and attach the lead wire from the iontophoresis unit that is the same polarity as the medication.

11. Apply the dispersive electrode (which is larger) to the muscle belly of a muscle approximately 2 to 3 inches away from the target treatment area. Ensure that the dispersive electrode is moist and also has good contact with the underlying skin. Connect the other lead wire to the dispersive electrode.

12. Follow the treatment protocols for the parameters of stimulation and slowly adjust the intensity. Remember that the intensity must not be greater than 1 mAmp/cm^2.

Intensity (mAmp)	Time (minutes)	Target
1	40	40 mAmp Minutes
2	20	40 mAmp Minutes
4	10	40 mAmp Minutes

13. Iontophoresis is applied with the patient in a comfortable, supported, neutral position.

14. Provide the patient with a means to contact you during the treatment time if needed. Remind the patient what to expect from the iontophoresis application and to let you know if it feels uncomfortable.

15. Re-check the patient after 3 to 5 minutes to ensure that he or she is still comfortable.

16. When the treatment time concludes, make sure the intensity is at zero. Remove the electrodes from the patient and check the skin for signs of irritation. Note any abnormal responses in the patient's chart.

17. It may be necessary to apply a moisturizer to the patient's skin where the electrodes were placed to help decrease irritation that occurred during stimulation.

18. Explain to the patient what he or she potentially could expect later in the day as a result of the application of iontophoresis.

1. Review the precautions and contraindications before applying hydrotherapy to ensure that its use is safe for this patient at this time.

2. Explain the modality to the patient so that he or she will know what to expect from the application of hydrotherapy.

3. Inspect the skin overlying the treatment area where hydrotherapy will be applied. Assess for blanching, increased temperature, and the presence of scars. If there are any irregularities not sufficient to cause a change in the treatment approach, note them in the patient's chart and continue with the application.

4. If a significant amount of the patient's body will be submersed in water, it would be appropriate to monitor the patient's vital signs before the application of the hydrotherapy. For example, if the patient will be going into a high-boy or low-boy tank, record the pretreatment blood pressure and heart rate. If the patient is having his or her upper extremity submersed, then this step would not be as necessary.

5. Fill the treatment tank with water that is an appropriate temperature according to the treatment goal for that patient.

6. Position the patient for the application of the hydrotherapy so that he or she is supported in a neutral position. For example, if the patient will be using an extremity tank, ensure that the seat is at an appropriate height for the patient and that there is a towel to pad him or her from the edge of the tank.

7. Remove the patient's clothing from the treatment area.

8. Place the treatment area in the tank, adjust the turbulence if indicated, and adjust the aeration if indicated.

9. Provide the patient with a means to contact you during the treatment time if needed. Remind the patient what to expect from the hydrotherapy application and to let you know if it feels uncomfortable.

10. Re-check the patient after 5 minutes to ensure that he or she is still comfortable.

11. When the treatment time concludes, remove the patient from the whirlpool and dry the area with a towel.

12. Check the area that was treated. Inspect the skin for normal and abnormal physiological responses. Note any abnormal responses in the patient's chart.

13. Empty the water from the tank and follow the department's protocol for cleaning the tank and turbine.

▰ AQUATIC THERAPY

1. Review the precautions and contraindications before applying aquatic therapy to ensure that its use is safe for this patient at this time.

2. Explain the modality to the patient so that he or she will know what to expect from the application of aquatic therapy.

3. Review the goals of aquatic therapy with the patient before entering the pool environment. Ask whether the patient has any questions or fears. Determine whether the patient can swim.

4. Advise the patient that he or she will be required to provide a bathing suit and will be showering before entering the pool. The patient also will be responsible for getting dressed after the aquatic therapy session and should come prepared with towels and a hair dryer. If assistance is needed to dress or undress or to otherwise prepare for the aquatic environment, these details should be worked out before the treatment session.

5. Assemble any flotation devices you will use with the patient during the aquatic therapy session so they are readily available and accessible.

6. Some clinicians prefer to wear wet suits in addition to a bathing suit for aquatic therapy sessions with patients. Decide this in advance, and have a wet suit available if you wish to use one.

7. Develop a plan to transfer the patient into the pool. This will be based on the facilities that are available, the needs of the patient, and the goals of the treatment session.

8. Monitor and record the patient's vital signs.

9. Help the patient transfer into the pool as needed.

10. Implement the treatment plan with the patient in the pool.

11. Monitor the patient's response to the aquatic environment throughout the treatment time. Some patients fatigue quickly in a buoyant environment; others chill quickly. Constant feedback from patients is critical for patient safety.

12. When the treatment session concludes, assist the patient as needed in transferring out of the water. Monitor his or her post-treatment vital signs

13. Assist the patient in drying off with towels and returning to the changing area as needed.

14. Document the treatment session time and activities performed, indicating those that were buoyancy assisted or buoyancy resisted. It is also useful to record patient responses to the session and post-treatment vital signs.

■ ELECTRICAL STIMULATION FOR PAIN RELIEF (TENS)

1. Review the precautions and contraindications before applying transcutaneous electrical nerve stimulation (TENS) to ensure that its use is safe for this patient at this time.

2. Inspect the lead wires to ensure that they are intact and there are no breaks in the protective outer covering surrounding the wires.

3. Select a TENS unit according to the needs of the patient.
   - One that has the appropriate parameters based upon the types discomfort the patient has and the modes of stimulation that you will use
   - One that has a variety of electrodes available to fit the needs of the patient

4. Select electrodes that are appropriate for the application based on the treatment area where you will apply them.

5. Explain the modality to the patient so that he or she will know what to expect from the application of TENS

6. Ask the patient to rate his or her discomfort on a scale of 1 to 10, with 1 representing no pain and 10 representing the worst pain possible. Record that number in the patient's chart.

7. Inspect the skin overlying the treatment area where TENS will be applied. Assess for blanching, increased temperature, the presence of scars, and absent or altered sensation. If there are any irregularities not sufficient to cause a change in the treatment approach, note them in the patient's chart and continue with the application.

8. Remove the patient's clothing in the treatment area and ensure adequate access.

9. Clean the skin before applying the electrodes, making sure that there are no lotions, oils, or anything else that might inhibit the uniform flow of electrical energy into the patient.

10. Prepare the electrodes for application to the patient according to the directions on the packaging. Moist electrode interfaces help to decrease the resistance to the flow of current and make the sensation more comfortable for the patient with less intensity.

11. Consult placement charts to determine where the electrodes should be applied according to the patient's complaints of discomfort.

12. TENS is applied in the clinic with the patient in a comfortable, supported, neutral position.

13. Apply the TENS electrodes to the patient making sure that there is good contact between the electrodes and the skin. It may be necessary to secure the electrodes with a strap to help conform them to the surface of the patient's affected body part.

14. Set the parameters according to the treatment goals and the level of disability of the patient.
    - Sensory analgesia: Short pulse duration and high frequency
    - Chronic pain syndromes: Long pulse duration and low frequency

15. Provide the patient with a means to contact you during the treatment time if needed. Remind the patient what to expect from the TENS application and to let you know if it feels uncomfortable.

16. Re-check the patient after 3 to 5 minutes to ensure that he or she is still comfortable. Ask the patient what he or she feels.
    - Parameters set for sensory analgesia:
        - If the response is "tingling," the electrode placement sites were appropriate.
        - If the response is "I still feel pain," the electrode placement sites may need to be adjusted.
    - Parameters set for chronic pain syndromes:
        - If the response is "I feel a thumping sensation," the stimulation is working properly. The patient probably will not feel any relief of symptoms for at least 20 minutes.
        - If the response is "I feel nothing," the intensity is not high enough. The batteries in the TENS unit may need to be replaced if a portable unit is being used.

17. When the treatment time concludes, remove the electrodes from the patient and check the skin for signs of irritation. Note any abnormal responses in the patient's chart.

18. Explain to the patient what he or she potentially could expect later in the day as a result of the application of TENS, including how the stimulated muscles might feel and what to do if the muscles feel fatigued.

19. Ask the patient to rate his or her discomfort using the scale described previously. Record that number in the patient's chart as a post-treatment pain rating.

◼ TRANSCUTANEOUS ELECTRICAL NERVE STIMULATION (TENS HOME UNIT)

1. Review the precautions and contraindications before applying transcutaneous electrical nerve stimulation (TENS) to ensure that its use is safe for this patient at this time.

2. Inspect the equipment's lead wires to ensure that they are intact and free of breaks in the protective outer covering surrounding the wires.

3. Ask the patient to rate his or her discomfort on a scale of 1 to 10, with 1 representing no pain and 10 representing the worst pain possible. Record that number in the patient's chart.

4. Select a TENS unit to meet the needs of the patient.
   - One that has the appropriate parameters based on the types discomfort the patient has and the modes of stimulation that you will use
   - One that accommodates the dexterity of the patient and his or her ability to adjust the intensity controls independently
   - One that has a trial TENS unit available for use to determine whether this will be the best unit for the patient before purchase
   - One that has a variety of electrodes available to fit the needs of the patient.

5. Select electrodes that are appropriate for the application based on the treatment area where they will be applied and the ready availability of replacements.

6. Explain the modality to the patient so that he or she will know what to expect from the application of TENS. Ensure the patient understands that he or she will have the ability to adjust the unit independently to control his or her discomfort during the day.

7. Inspect the skin overlying the treatment area where TENS will be applied. Assess for blanching, increased temperature, the presence of scars, and absent or altered sensation. If there are any irregularities not sufficient to cause a change in the treatment approach, note them in the patient's chart and continue with the application.

8. Adjust the patient's clothing to ensure access to the treatment area. It is not necessary to remove the patient's clothing to apply the electrodes. The patient will be able to apply the electrodes and wear the unit under his or her clothing during the day.

9. Explain the process and importance of cleaning the skin before applying the electrodes, making sure that there are no lotions, oils, or anything else that might inhibit the uniform flow of electrical energy into the patient.

10. Help the patient prepare the electrodes for application according to the directions on the packaging. Moist electrode interfaces help to decrease the resistance to the flow of current and make the sensation more comfortable for the patient with less intensity. This must be explained to the patient in simple terms.

11. Consult placement charts to determine where the electrodes should be applied according to the patient's complaints of discomfort.

12. TENS is usually applied in the clinic with the patient positioned in a comfortable, supported, neutral position. However, home TENS units are designed to be worn underneath clothing and adjusted when discomfort is perceived.

13. Assist the patient in applying the TENS electrodes to the patient making sure that there is good contact between the electrodes and the skin.

14. Help the patient position his or her clothing so that the lead wires of the TENS unit are hidden.

15. Set the parameters according to the treatment goals and the level of disability of the patient. Explain the adjustments to the patient and have him or her adjust these settings.
    - Sensory analgesia: Short pulse duration and high frequency
    - Chronic pain syndromes: Long pulse duration and low frequency

16. Stay with the patient while he or she adjusts the intensity of the TENS unit to ensure that he or she understands what to expect from the stimulation.

17. Provide the patient with a means to contact you during the treatment time if needed. Remind the patient what to expect from the TENS application and to let you know if it feels uncomfortable.

18. Re-check the patient after 3 to 5 minutes to ensure that he or she is still comfortable. Ask the patient what he or she feels.
    - Parameters set for sensory analgesia:
        - If the response is "tingling," the electrode placement sites were appropriate.
        - If the response is "I still feel pain," the electrode placement sites may need to be adjusted.
    - Parameters set for chronic pain syndromes:
        - If the response is "I feel a thumping sensation," the stimulation is working properly. The patient probably will not feel any relief of symptoms for at least 20 minutes.
        - If the response is "I feel nothing," the intensity is not high enough. The batteries in the TENS unit may need to be replaced.

19. When the treatment time concludes, instruct the patient in how to remove the electrodes and check the skin for signs of irritation. Note any abnormal responses in the patient's chart.

20. Explain what the patient could potentially expect later in the day as a result of the application TENS and how the stimulated muscles might feel and what to do if the muscles do feel fatigued.

21. Ask the patient to rate his or her discomfort according to the scale described previously. Record that number in the patient's chart as a post-treatment pain rating. Ask the patient to keep a log of pretreatment and post-treatment pain ratings. Also have them note how long the relief lasts before the patient feels the need to turn on the TENS unit again.

22. Instruct the patient in the proper removal of the electrodes and care of the lead wires and electrodes. Also be sure to instruct the patient in the location and removal and replacement of the battery from the TENS unit.

23. Provide the patient with a written set of instructions that include everything you discussed orally regarding the application of the TENS unit and how to set the parameters. Be sure to include illustrations of the electrode placement sites indicating which electrodes should be set up on each channel.

THERAPEUTIC ULTRASOUND

1. Review the precautions and contraindications before applying ultrasound to ensure that its use is safe for this patient at this time.

2. Explain the modality to the patient so that he or she will know what to expect from the application of ultrasound.

3. Inspect the skin overlying the treatment area where ultrasound will be applied. Assess for blanching, increased temperature, and the presence of scars. If there are any irregularities not sufficient to cause a change in the treatment approach, note them in the patient's chart and continue with the application.

4. Position the patient for the application of the ultrasound so that he or she is supported in a neutral position. For example, for treatment of the lumbar spine, the patient should be treated prone with a pillow under the lumbar spine and ankles. Treatment of the cervical muscles should also occur supine or prone with pillows for support to allow the postural muscles to be unloaded.

5. Ask yourself the following questions about the patient to help determine the treatment parameters for the application of ultrasound.
   - Is the target treatment tissue superficial or deep?
     - Superficial: 3 MHz
     - Deep: 1 MHz
   - Is the condition acute or chronic? The more acute the condition, the lower the duty factor should be.
   - Is there a significant amount of or very little soft tissue in the treatment area? If there is not much soft tissue in the treatment area, it is safer to start with a lower intensity (W/cm2).
   - How large is the treatment area, and how large is the transducer? The treatment area should not be more than twice the size of the transducer.
   - Treatment times should equal 2 minutes per treatment area equal to the size of the transducer when continuous ultrasound is being applied. Treatment times may need to be adjusted for pulsed ultrasound applications to accommodate for total energy delivered to the patient.
   - Set all of the parameters except the intensity.
   - Document the parameters in the patient's chart.

6. Remove the patient's clothing from the treatment area.

7. Palpate the treatment area to determine whether there are any specific areas within a muscle that have a fibrocystic component; these often respond well to ultrasound. Ask the patient to rate his or her discomfort when identified areas are palpated. Record patient responses to palpation as pretreatment findings and note the locations for treatment.

8. Apply a small amount of acoustically conductive lotion or gel to the surface of the ultrasound transducer, enough to cover the surface of the transducer.

9. Inform the patient that you will be touching him or her with the transducer, which might feel cool. Apply the transducer to the patient. Set the intensity and move the transducer to treat the patient with ultrasound.

10. Remind the patient what to expect during ultrasound treatment and to let you know if he or she feels anything uncomfortable. If the patient reports feeling a burning sensation, move the transducer more quickly (speed should be approximately 1 cm/sec) or decrease the intensity.

11. The transducer must be kept moving during the treatment time, and you must also continuously ensure that there is good contact between the transducer and the patient's skin. Avoid the temptation to lift the head of the transducer to re-capture the acoustical media.

12. When the treatment time concludes, remove the transducer from the patient, wipe off the gel or lotion, and carefully place it back in its cradle in the ultrasound unit. Then wipe the gel or lotion from the patient with a towel and inspect the treatment area

13. Re-palpate the area that was treated with the ultrasound, noting any changes in the soft tissue and the patient's response to that palpation compared with the pre-treatment palpation. Document the patient's post-treatment responses to palpation and your post-treatment palpation findings.

◼ HOT PACKS

1. Review the precautions and contraindications before applying a hot pack to ensure that its use is safe for this patient at this time.

2. Explain the modality to the patient so that he or she will know what to expect from the application of the hot pack.

3. Inspect the skin overlying the treatment area where the hot pack will be applied. Assess for blanching, increased temperature, and the presence of scars. If there are any irregularities not sufficient to cause a change in the treatment approach, note them in the patient's chart and continue with the application.

4. Position the patient for the application of the hot pack so that he or she is supported in a neutral position. For example, for treatment of the lumbar spine, the patient should be treated prone with a pillow placed under the lumbar spine and ankles. Treatment of the cervical muscles should also occur with the patient supine or prone and supported by pillows to allow the postural muscles to be unloaded.

5. Remove the patient's clothing over the treatment area and apply sufficient layers of toweling so that the hot pack covered in the commercial cover will touch the patient's skin. There should be no clothing between the hot pack and the patient's skin.

6. Apply the hot pack to the patient making sure that there is good contact between the hot pack and the skin. It may be necessary to secure the hot pack with an additional towel layer to help conform it to the surface of the patient's affected body part.

7. Drape the patient so that no skin is exposed.

8. Provide the patient with a means to contact you during the treatment time if needed. Remind the patient what to expect from the hot pack application and to let you know if it feels uncomfortable.

9. Re-check the patient after 3 to 5 minutes to ensure that he or she is still comfortable. This is when the hot pack will reach peak temperature, and the patient might need additional layers of toweling.

10. When the treatment time concludes, remove the hot pack from the patient but leave one layer of toweling over the treatment area while you return the hot pack to the hot pack unit. This layer of toweling is warm and will keep the area warm until you return.

11. Check the area that was treated with the hot pack. Inspect the skin for normal and abnormal physiological responses to the hot pack. Note any abnormal responses in the patient's chart.

12. Return the hot pack to the heating unit. It will take approximately 30 minutes before the hot pack is reheated sufficiently to be used for another patient. Hang the commercial cover to dry.

CRYOTHERAPY

1. Review the precautions and contraindications before applying cryotherapy to ensure that its use is safe for this patient at this time.

2. Explain the modality to the patient so that he or she will know what to expect from the application of the cryotherapy.

3. Inspect the skin overlying the treatment area where cryotherapy will be applied. Assess for blanching, increased temperature, and the presence of scars. If there are any irregularities not sufficient to cause a change in the treatment approach, note them in the patient's chart and continue with the application.

4. Position the patient for the application of cryotherapy so that he or she is supported in a neutral position.
   - If you are using ice massage, ensure that you have a towel under the area to catch melted ice, as this is uncomfortable for the patient.
   - If you are applying an ice pack to the cervical spine, ensure that the patient is either supine or prone to unload the cervical musculature.
   - If you are applying cryotherapy using an ice bath, ensure that the patient can sit in a comfortable position during the application.

5. Remove the patient's clothing from the treatment area.
   - Ice massage must be applied directly to the patient's skin.
   - There should be no clothing between the cold pack and the patient's skin. Follow the procedures set by the facility regarding the placement of a paper towel or pillow case between the cold pack and the patient to maintain sanitary standards.
   - Ensure that all patient clothing is clear of the ice bath and does not accidentally slip into the ice bath during treatment.

6. Apply the selected form of cryotherapy to the patient.
   - If you are applying a cold pack, ensure that there is good contact between the cold pack and the patient's skin. It may be necessary to secure the cold pack with an additional towel layer to help the pack conform to the surface of the patient.

7. If you have selected a cold pack application, drape the patient so that no additional skin is exposed.

8. If you have selected a cold pack or ice bath, provide the patient with a means to contact you during the treatment time if needed. Remind the patient what to expect from the cold pack or ice bath application. It is common to first feel cold, then aching or burning, followed by numbness.

9. If you have selected a cold pack or ice bath, re-check the patient after 3 to 5 minutes to ensure that he or she is still comfortable. This is when the cryotherapy will reach the burning or aching phase, and the patient may need reassurance or repositioning.

10. If you have selected an ice massage, the treatment area must be small. Cover the ice with a paper towel so that your fingers are not directly touching the ice. The treatment area should not exceed 1 square inch, otherwise numbness will not be accomplished. Ask the patient for feedback regarding the stages of sensations that he or she is feeling to guide the length of the treatment time.

11. If you have selected a cold pack or ice bath, when the treatment time concludes, remove the patient from the ice bath or the cold pack from the patient. Dry the area with the towel.

12. Check the area that was treated with cryotherapy. Inspect the skin for normal and abnormal physiological responses to the treatment. Note any abnormal responses in the patient's chart.

13. Return the cold pack to the freezer. It will take approximately 30 minutes before the cold pack is re-cooled sufficiently to be used for another patient.